The Family Guide *to*
Reflexology

Ann Gillanders

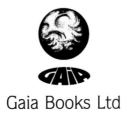

Gaia Books Ltd

A Gaia Original

Books from Gaia celebrate the vision of Gaia, the self-sustaining living Earth, and seek to help their readers live in greater personal and planetary harmony.

Editor Anne Kilborn

Designer Phil Gamble

Illustration Johanna Amos

Photography Annie Johnston

Managing Editor Pip Morgan

Production Lyn Kirby

Direction Patrick Nugent

Consultant Dr Helen Dziemidko

This book is not intended to replace medical care under the direct supervision of a qualified doctor. Before embarking on any changes in your health regime, consult your doctor.

First published in the United Kingdom in 1998 by
Gaia Books Ltd, 66 Charlotte St, London W1P 1LR
and 20 High St, Stroud, Glos GL5 1AS

ISBN 1 85675 049 3

A catalogue record of this book is available from the British Library.

Printed and bound in Singapore by Kyodo

10 9 8 7 6 5 4 3 2 1

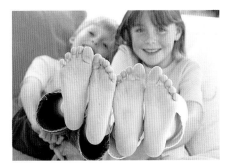

Contents

Introduction

"Hands are made for healing, and the healing power of touch lies at all our fingertips. You only have to use it!"

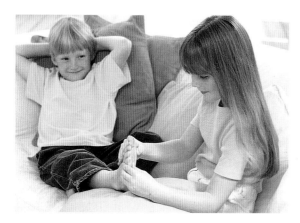

Loving family bonds *are strengthened through the healing power of touch. The demonstration of tender loving care through work on the feet helps build self-esteem and confidence as well as sensitivity toward others – in both giver and receiver.*

Since I began practising reflexology in 1974, I have given more than 35,000 treatments and trained many hundreds of therapists. I have treated people of all ages, from all walks of life, with all manner of ailments, and I have witnessed, time and again, the wonderful healing power of reflexology. Today, I find myself treating the children, and even the grandchildren, of people whom I treated when they themselves were much younger. This close involvement over many years with the progress of so many different families who turned to reflexology as a natural healing tool persuaded me of the need for a practical family guide that would enable others to enjoy its benefits.

From my own experience, I know that most everyday ailments can be relieved, and in many cases the symptoms removed altogether, by frequent reflexology treatments by a professional. Even more important, I have observed that reflexology has the power to promote and nourish an ongoing state of wellbeing. Regular treatments were part of our family routine and I am certain that it was because of them that my own children literally bounded with vitality and good health. What I prized above all, however, were the special times it

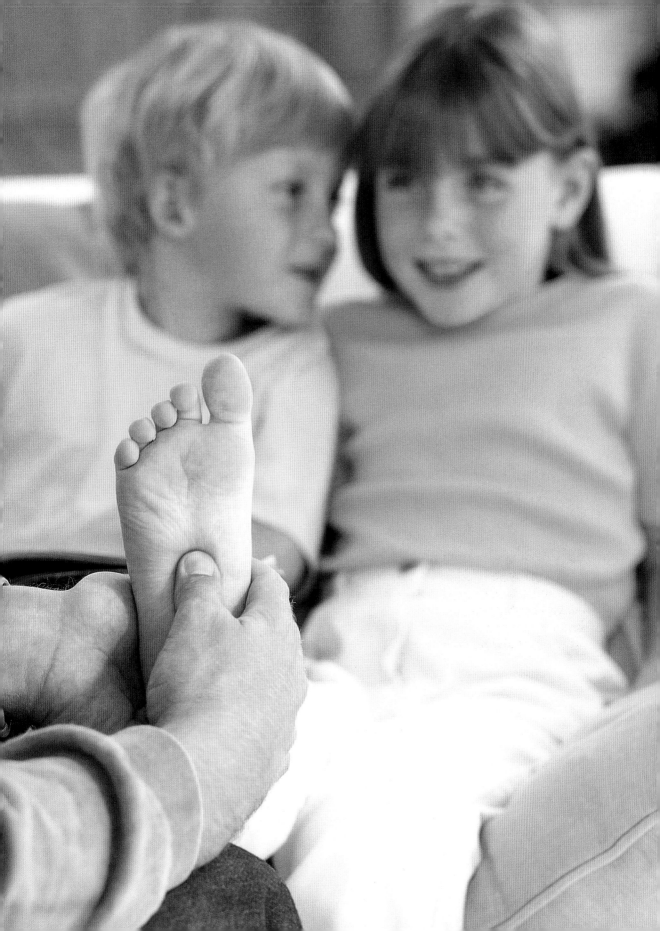

allowed me to devote myself individually to each of my four children. If time was short, I would simply give them the foot relaxing treatment. I still treasure the memory of these moments, when loving family bonds were reinforced through the healing power of touch.

First steps to family fitness

This volume, then, is intended as a practical manual for people who want to benefit, as a family, from all that reflexology has to offer.

While frequent treatments by a professional are clearly indicated in certain conditions, practical or financial considerations make it impossible for most people to seek professional help with the frequency their particular case demands.

In such instances, other family members often ask for guidance on offering the patient interim treatments at home. And when they give treatments on a regular basis there is no doubt that their supplementary efforts play an essential role in a successful outcome.

You will find reflexology beneficial for all generations, from the cradle onward. Indeed, it may be given immediately after their delivery to babies who suffered a traumatic birth, perhaps through forceps delivery or a prolonged labour.

I have included only those common ailments that I know respond well to treatments. Turn to the chapter on "Healthy Babies and Children" for advice on alleviating common conditions in the early years, including those with a strong stress component. So preoccupied are most adults with their own stress levels, they tend often to overlook the numerous stress-inducing situations their children are subjected to, often on a daily basis. At the same time they may fail to connect certain physical

symptoms – over-eating, bedwetting or being accident-prone – with an emotional cause.

"Treating Adult Ailments" (Chapter Four) is an easy-to-use practical guide to treating a number of common adult ailments. They are presented according to the area of the body in which they occur, and the chapter works from top (the head area) to toe. Open the page at the ailment you wish to treat and all you need to know to give an immediate treatment is in front of you. (This presupposes, of course, that you have already read and inwardly digested Chapter One where I explain the general basic principles and techniques of working.) The chapter concludes with advice on treating allergies and arthritis, both of which can affect a number of different areas of the body.

In Chapter Five, "Making Stress Manageable," I have discussed a number of life events and situations that are generally recognized as inducing a high level of stress, which reflexology treatments can, to some extent, relieve. Indeed, one of the major benefits of reflexology is its wonderfully relaxing effect, and if it were to work on this level and no other, its contribution to reducing stress and increasing resistance to "dis-ease", would be inestimable.

Reflexology can do more than this, however. There are numerous specific reflex points that can be worked to minimize the effects of stress-related conditions. You can help restore the sex drive by working the sexual reflexes in people whose interest is depleted; you can work the endocrine system to help restore hormonal balance in people who are depressed.

When you are part of a family, even the most personal problems are unlikely to be limited in their effect. Children, spouses, parents – all are eventually affected in some way or another by the dis-ease of one of their number. A common recognition of a problem and a united effort to deal with it as a family must be beneficial for everyone concerned. Reflexology is the ideal medium for expressing concern, and every family member can participate in it.

Reflexology, while producing many extraordinary results, is not, however, the ultimate panacea. It does not propose cures, it merely enables the body's own self-healing mechanism to function as best it can. And here it is important to consider the causes of the energy blockages that reflexology sets out to clear. Sometimes they are only too apparent: poor diet, over-indulgence (of one form or another), lack of exercise, an unhappy partnership, a frustrating or unsatisfying work situation – are some common causes.

If healing is to take place, I am now utterly convinced, the patient has to want to get better. In this respect, certain lifestyle changes may be necessary, to contribute toward recovery and restoration of balance. For this reason I have included throughout the book "support strategies" that can be used in conjunction with reflexology treatments. Most frequently mentioned, not surprisingly, are healthy eating and regular exercise, but relaxation and meditation, yoga, massage, aromatherapy, herbal, and traditional folk remedies also play an important role. Chapter Two is a basic introduction to some of these.

The joy of reflexology is in the opportunity it gives members of a family to express to one another how much they really care – with no need for words. The importance of this, particularly in families where physical contact is not part and parcel of everyday living, cannot be overestimated. If reflexology is an accepted part of their family life, children learn that the health and happiness of other members of the family really is their concern, and something in which they can play a vital role. This nurtures qualities of caring and responsibility that they will carry with them into adult life.

I have included a handful of case histories in this book. I could have cited many more. Those I have chosen are simply there to "bring alive" for you the benefits of reflexology for people of all ages.

Hands are made for healing, and the healing power of touch lies at all our fingertips. You only have to use it.

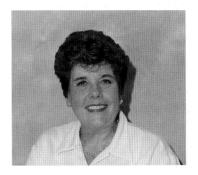

Ann Gillanders

Ann Gillanders
is Principal of the British School of Reflexology.

Chapter One

Releasing Blocked Energy

Using the thumb or forefinger to apply fine, deep pressure to appropriate reflex points, you can remove blockages in energy pathways and open the channels for natural healing.

When we went barefoot, padding over soft sand that moulded itself with every step to the contours of our feet, tip-toeing over forest floors or racing over grassy plains in pursuit of prey, shinning up trees in search of fruits, clambering over boulders, or wading across stony river beds, at every moment our feet were making contact with the healing earth. Yielding or unyielding, the ground was continually massaging the soles of our feet, sustaining the tremendous clear flow of energy necessary in the struggle for survival.

But that was long ago. Few people today in the western world ever abandon some form of footwear, except at night, and the surface we mostly tread is a smooth concrete carapace that separates us from the soil of our planet. Yet our feet still cry out for contact with the earth and, when we can, we still rejoice in running barefoot. When we return from a hard day's trek in the concrete jungle, we collapse in an armchair and throw off our shoes with sighs of relief. If a kindly relative then offers us a foot massage, our gratitude knows no bounds!

The pleasurable, therapeutic benefits of massaging both the feet and the hands have long been recognized. There is evidence that compression massage on the feet was used as long as 5,000 years ago in China. In ancient India and Egypt, too, manipulating particular points on the feet was known to have a healing effect. A frieze in the Physician's Tomb at Saqqara in Egypt depicts patients receiving both foot and hand treatments: it is more than 4,000 years old.

Channelling the life force
Though there is considerable evidence of reflexology having been used over the centuries in the western world, it only really "took off" in early nineteenth-century America, thanks to the efforts of Dr William Fitzgerald. This pioneer and popularizer of "zone therapy" inspired the physiotherapist Eunice Ingham whose patient and painstaking research led to the detailed maps of the feet with which any student of reflexology today is familiar.

Fitzgerald had divided the body into 10 energy zones, 5 on each side of the spine,

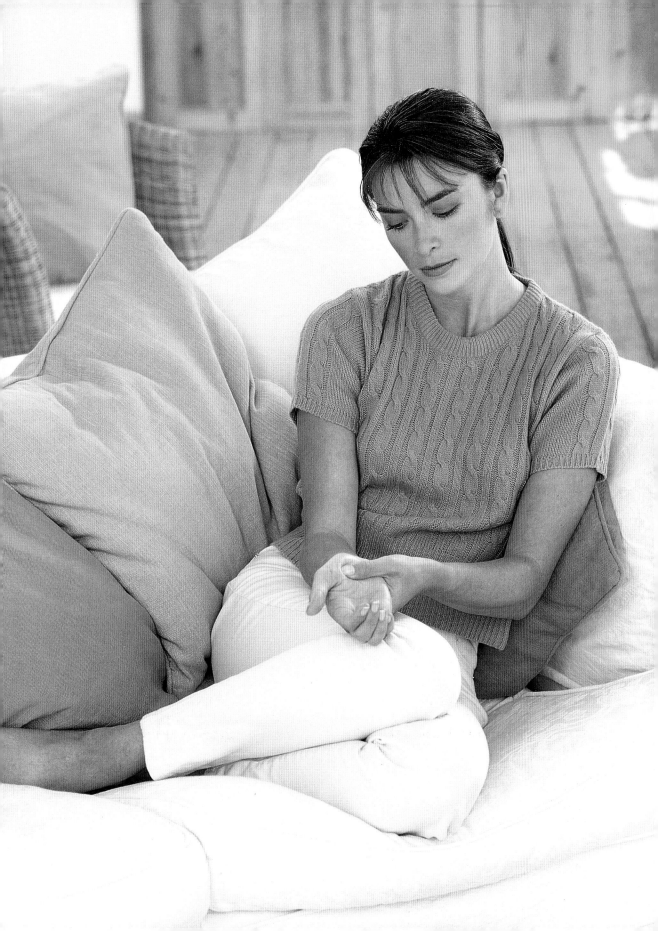

running from the big toe (zone 1) up through the head. The hands are zoned, with zone 1 starting at the thumbs. Not only do these zones run longitudinally, they pass through the body, from back to front.

Restoring harmony and balance

All the organs, muscles, and functions of the body lie in one or more of these zones, and their corresponding reflexes are found in the same zones on the feet and hands. Each zone is a channel for the life force, known as "chi" to the Chinese, "prana" to Hindus, and any obstruction or blockage in that energy flow affects the organs or functions within it, leading to dis-ease.

Such obstructions, according to modern reflexologists, are caused by "crystalline" calcium deposits on delicate nerve endings, due to congestion, inflammation, or tension in the nerve pathways. Pressure on the reflexes, which encompass minute nerve complexes, breaks down these deposits, and frees the pathways.

Thus, by applying pressure to reflex points, the reflexologist eventually releases blocked energy, restoring a clear flow throughout the body. This is the first step toward restoring harmony and balance – a first step in the healing process.

The reflex maps

It is not necessary to know a great deal more about the zones. More important are the maps of the feet and hands, which you need to consult in order to locate the reflexes related to specific organs and areas of the body. The original foot maps were devised by Eunice Ingham, who realized that the most effective way of working on energy channels was through the feet. While William Fitzgerald had worked on the fingers, mainly to produce local anesthetic

effects, she recognized the wider therapeutic benefits of work on the energy zones. She concentrated her attention on the feet because they are extremely sensitive, with more than 7,000 nerve endings, and eventually produced detailed maps showing which part of the foot to work in order to clear the energy channels for particular parts of the body.

The maps on pp. 14-19 are the author's own and incorporate changes and amendments to Ingham's originals, based on her own working experience and observations over many years.

The position of the reflexes on the soles of the feet mirrors their arrangement in the body. This is clear if you imagine the sole maps next to each other, with the spine running down the middle, and the toes representing the head. Working down toward the heel, you come to the chest area (with lungs, heart, and, on the outside, the shoulders), the stomach area (with the stomach and organs associated with digestion), and below it the intestines.

The right foot maps the right side of the body and the left foot, the left side. The symmetry of external body parts on either side of the spine is reflected in identical reflex points on both right and left feet. While certain internal organs are also identical on both, asymmetry is evident in the heart (mainly on the left side) and the reflexes to the liver (mainly on the left) and the stomach (on the right).

Working guidelines

These lines divide the feet and hands into broad sections that mirror "divisions" of the body. As you would expect, then, the areas of the head, neck, and shoulders, as well as the heart and lungs, lie above the diaphragm line. On the feet the diaphragm line is easy to identify because the skin just above it is darker in colour than that below. On the hands, it is about 2.5cm (1in) below the point where the index finger joins the hand.

The waist line is approximately in the middle of the foot. Identify it by running your finger down the outside edge of the foot until you come across a small bone that sticks out – the metatarsal notch. A line drawn straight across the foot at this point would represent the waist line. On the hands, the waist line runs across from the point where the thumb joins the hand. Between the waist line and the diaphragm line lie the organs of digestion, including the stomach and pancreas on the left foot, the liver on the right.

The pelvic line on the foot can be isolated by placing your index fingers on the patient's ankle bones and imagining a line drawn between them. On the hands, the pelvic line begins about 2.5cm (1in) down from the wrist, on the soft, fleshy pad of the thumb. Between the pelvic and waist lines lie the organs of elimination. Below the pelvic line are the sexual and reproductive areas.

The shoulder line, a secondary guideline, is located only on the feet, just below the base of the toes.

You can identify the ligament line by pulling back the toes to stretch the skin over the arch. You will feel the ligament just below the surface in a line between the first and second toes. The ligament line on the hands starts between the second and third fingers. Take care when working the feet not to apply pressure directly on the ligament line, since it is very tender.

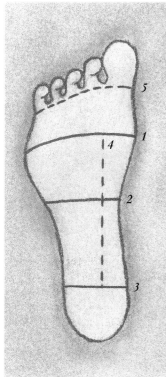

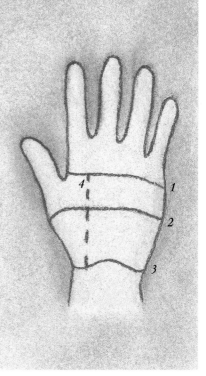

Working guidelines
These broad horizontal divisions of the soles of the feet and the palms of the hands are an essential adjunct to mapping your working territory. Memorize them and use them in conjunction with the maps on pp. 14-19 to locate and treat the reflexes above, below, or inbetween them.

1 Diaphragm line
2 Waist line
3 Pelvic line
4 Ligament line
5 Shoulder line (foot only)

The sole maps
The right foot

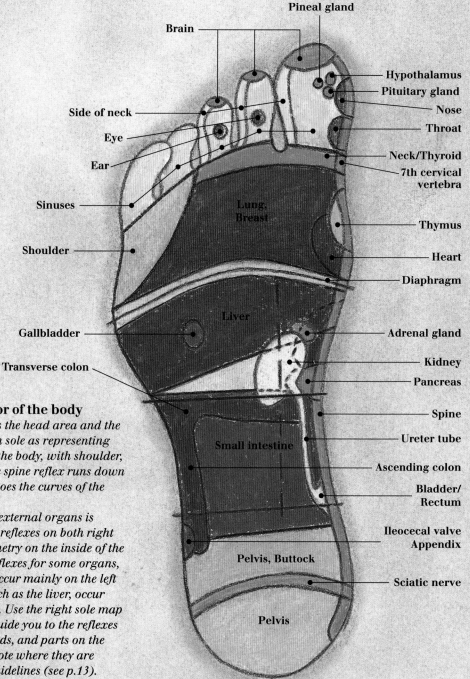

Pineal gland
Brain
Hypothalamus
Pituitary gland
Side of neck
Nose
Eye
Throat
Ear
Neck/Thyroid
7th cervical vertebra
Sinuses
Lung, Breast
Thymus
Shoulder
Heart
Diaphragm
Liver
Gallblader
Adrenal gland
Transverse colon
Kidney
Pancreas
Spine
Ureter tube
Small intestine
Ascending colon
Bladder/Rectum
Ileocecal valve Appendix
Pelvis, Buttock
Sciatic nerve
Pelvis

The feet: a mirror of the body

Visualize the toes as the head area and the outside edge of each sole as representing the outside edge of the body, with shoulder, waist, and hips. The spine reflex runs down the middle, and echoes the curves of the spine itself.

The symmetry of external organs is evident in identical reflexes on both right and left feet. Asymmetry on the inside of the body means that reflexes for some organs, such as the heart, occur mainly on the left foot while some, such as the liver, occur mainly on the right. Use the right sole map (plantar view) to guide you to the reflexes for all organs, glands, and parts on the right of the body. Note where they are in relation to the guidelines (see p.13).

The left foot

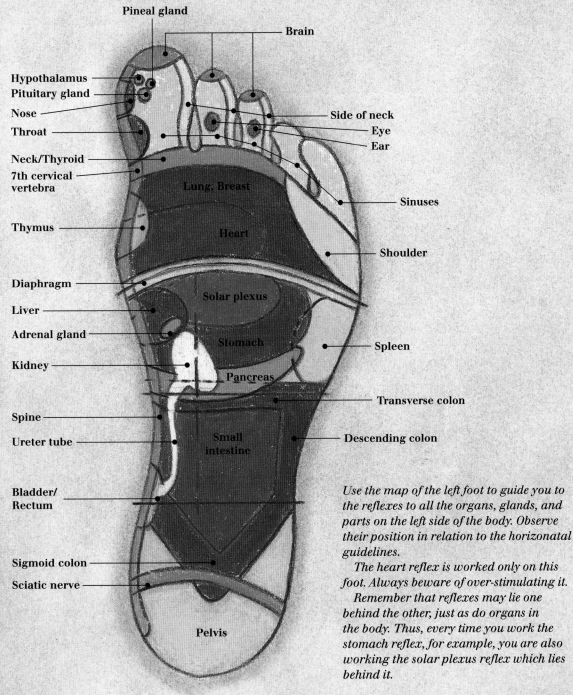

Pineal gland

Brain

Hypothalamus

Pituitary gland

Nose

Throat

Neck/Thyroid

7th cervical vertebra

Side of neck

Eye

Ear

Lung, Breast

Heart

Sinuses

Thymus

Shoulder

Diaphragm

Solar plexus

Liver

Adrenal gland

Stomach

Spleen

Kidney

Pancreas

Transverse colon

Spine

Ureter tube

Small intestine

Descending colon

Bladder/ Rectum

Sigmoid colon

Sciatic nerve

Pelvis

Use the map of the left foot to guide you to the reflexes to all the organs, glands, and parts on the left side of the body. Observe their position in relation to the horizonatal guidelines.

The heart reflex is worked only on this foot. Always beware of over-stimulating it.

Remember that reflexes may lie one behind the other, just as do organs in the body. Thus, every time you work the stomach reflex, for example, you are also working the solar plexus reflex which lies behind it.

The top and side maps

The right foot

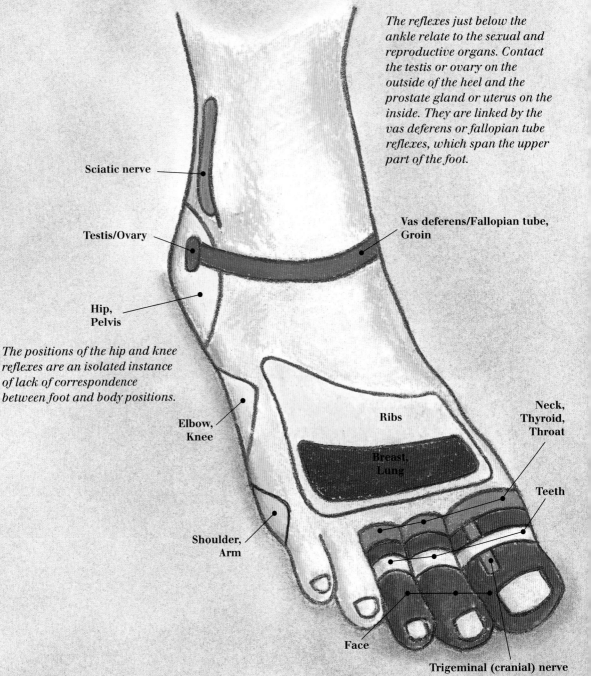

The reflexes just below the ankle relate to the sexual and reproductive organs. Contact the testis or ovary on the outside of the heel and the prostate gland or uterus on the inside. They are linked by the vas deferens or fallopian tube reflexes, which span the upper part of the foot.

Sciatic nerve

Testis/Ovary

Vas deferens/Fallopian tube, Groin

Hip, Pelvis

The positions of the hip and knee reflexes are an isolated instance of lack of correspondence between foot and body positions.

Elbow, Knee

Ribs

Neck, Thyroid, Throat

Breast, Lung

Teeth

Shoulder, Arm

Face

Trigeminal (cranial) nerve

The left foot

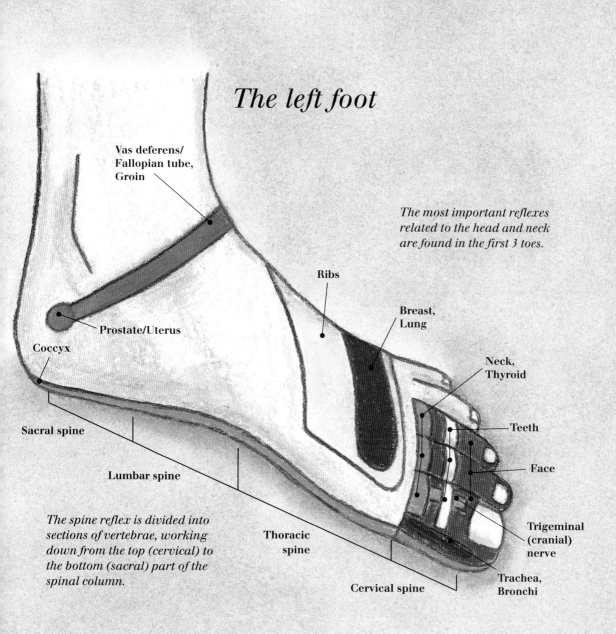

Vas deferens/
Fallopian tube,
Groin

*The most important reflexes
related to the head and neck
are found in the first 3 toes.*

Ribs

Breast,
Lung

Prostate/Uterus

Coccyx

Neck,
Thyroid

Sacral spine

Teeth

Face

Lumbar spine

*The spine reflex is divided into
sections of vertebrae, working
down from the top (cervical) to
the bottom (sacral) part of the
spinal column.*

Thoracic
spine

Trigeminal
(cranial)
nerve

Cervical spine

Trachea,
Bronchi

The maps for the tops and sides of the feet are far
simpler than those for the soles.

On the outside (lateral) edge of each foot, the
reflex points correspond roughly with the outer
sides of the body. However the relative positions
of hip and knee reflexes are unexpected, with the
knee coming between the shoulder and the hip.
This is an isolated instance of the nerve pathways
and their reflex points not corresponding with the

position of the prime body part. The top (or dorsal)
part of the foot has few reflexes: it is too bony to
allow effective contact. Note, however, that it is
the main part to contact for the breast reflex. This
shares its reflex with the lung, which is contacted
mainly on the sole of the foot.

The important spine reflex runs along the inside
edge of each foot, the curves of which echo those
of the spine itself.

The hand maps

All the reflex points relating to parts, glands, and organs in the body are found on the hands and wrists as well as the feet. Because of the smaller size of the hand, and the separation between fingers and thumb, the layout is more compressed, and less obvious than on the feet. The colour codes on the foot maps are repeated here on the hands.

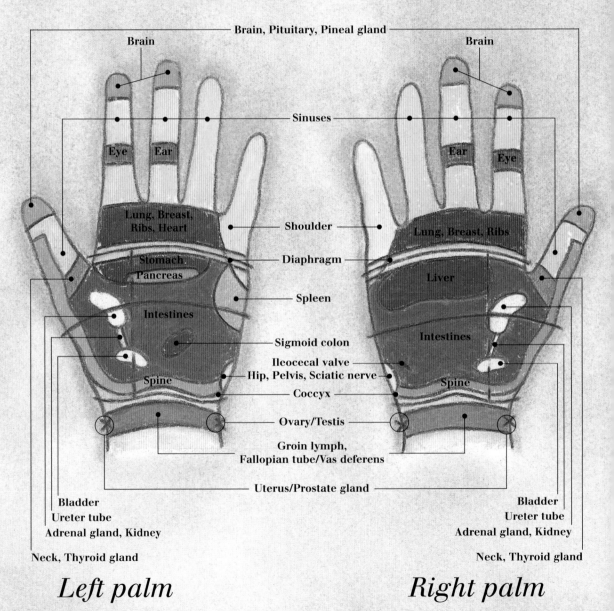

Brain, Pituitary, Pineal gland

Brain

Brain

Sinuses

Eye   Ear

Ear   Eye

Lung, Breast, Ribs, Heart

Shoulder

Lung, Breast, Ribs

Stomach
Pancreas

Diaphragm

Liver

Spleen

Intestines

Intestines

Sigmoid colon

Ileocecal valve

Spine

Hip, Pelvis, Sciatic nerve

Spine

Coccyx

Ovary/Testis

Groin lymph,
Fallopian tube/Vas deferens

Uterus/Prostate gland

Bladder
Ureter tube
Adrenal gland, Kidney

Bladder
Ureter tube
Adrenal gland, Kidney

Neck, Thyroid gland

Neck, Thyroid gland

Left palm

Right palm

Certain reflex points "wrap around" from the palm to the tops of the hands, some forming "rings" or "bracelets" around fingers and wrists. Thus maps of the sides of the hands are unnecessary.

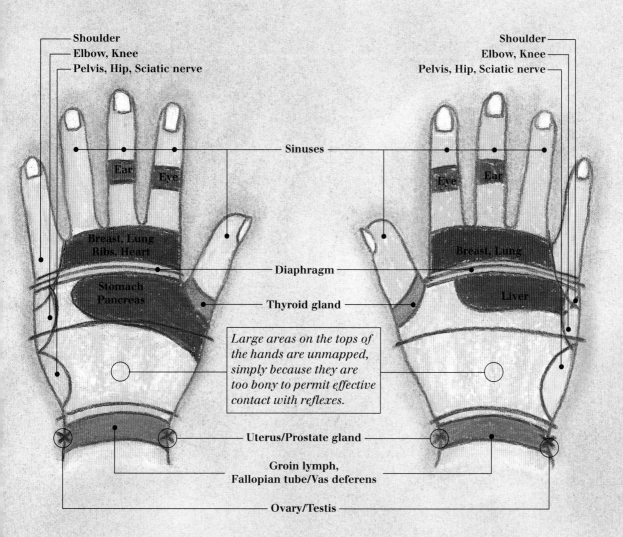

Shoulder
Elbow, Knee
Pelvis, Hip, Sciatic nerve

Shoulder
Elbow, Knee
Pelvis, Hip, Sciatic nerve

Sinuses

Ear
Eye

Eye
Ear

Breast, Lung
Ribs, Heart

Breast, Lung

Diaphragm

Stomach
Pancreas

Thyroid gland

Liver

Large areas on the tops of the hands are unmapped, simply because they are too bony to permit effective contact with reflexes.

Uterus/Prostate gland

Groin lymph,
Fallopian tube/Vas deferens

Ovary/Testis

Top of left hand

Top of right hand

Contacting the reflexes

When you first begin giving reflexology treatments, you will probably find that you are "all thumbs."You simply cannot get them to work with a smooth, consistent pressure: at one moment you are "digging in" to the foot, at the next you are skating over it. Take heart: the more you practise, as with anything else, the more accomplished you become. Aim, eventually, to use both thumbs and both forefingers with equal ease. Do not, in the meantime, resort to using oils or creams to smooth your path: it is impossible to contact reflex points when the skin is slippery. You may, however, use a light dusting of baby powder if you wish.

There are thousands of reflex points on the soles of the feet and the palms of the hands. Your aim is to apply pressure to as many as possible in the appropriate area, using either your thumb or forefinger. In order to get an idea of how small the movements should be, envisage the reflex points (which are no bigger than a pinhead) as pins densely packed in a plump, old-fashioned pincushion. Imagine that you are firmly pressing one pin after the other down into the cushion, always working in a forward direction.This technique is used to give most of the treatments recommended in this book.

When treating very small areas (on the toes, for example), just rotate the thumb or finger clockwise on the spot, or alternately apply and then release pressure.Support the top of the foot if you are treating areas above the waist line (see p. 13); support the heel if you are working below it. Tension in your hands is felt by the receiver, so hold the foot , neither too firmly nor too lightly.

Be sensitive to sensitivities

Adjust the pressure you apply according to the person you are treating. A gentle pressure is appropriate for babies, young children, and older people. A firm pressure is called for in most other cases. Keep an eye on the receiver's facial expression: it will alert you to sensitive spots. Once aware of discomfort, reduce the pressure immediately.

How to use your thumbs and fingers

Keep your thumb (or finger) flexed as in the drawing – neither too arched, nor too flat. Do not keep straightening and flexing it. Work with the flat pad of the thumb, pressing down slightly on the outer edge, so that the flesh folds back to provide a protective barrier against the nail.

Edge or "creep" forward in minute stages, as if pressing pins into a pincushion. Maintaining permanent contact with the skin, work slowly and methodically over the appropriate area.

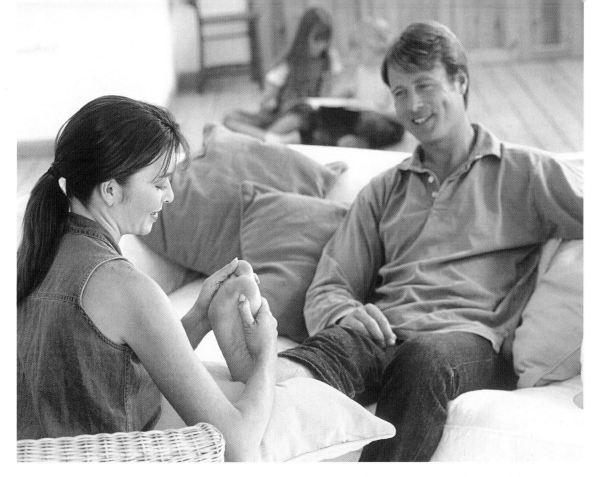

For the treatment to be successful, it is essential that both of you are sitting comfortably. Physical discomfort is translated into tension, which interrupts the energy flow and impedes healing.

A suitable place for treatment

You will both enjoy the session more if it takes place in pleasant surroundings where you are unlikely to be interrupted. Flowers always enhance a room, and if you think it appropriate, you could play some relaxing music as a background to treatment. Before starting make sure your hands are clean and nails trimmed.

Sit the receiver in a comfortable armchair or garden lounger, perhaps with a stool to support the leg. Seat yourself at a suitable height, facing the receiver so that you can "read" their facial expression. Rest the foot to be treated on a cushion in your lap.

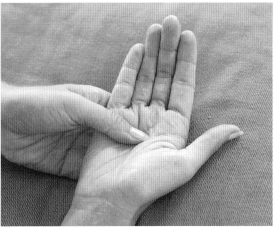

When working your own hands, it may be more comfortable to rest the hand you are treating on a small cushion in your lap. Use a little talcum powder on the hands if you wish, but, as with the feet, do not use oils that make the skin slippery and contact with the reflex points difficult.

Basic principles of treatment

Reflexology is a holistic therapy, and for this reason it is always preferable to treat the whole person by treating the whole foot (or the whole hand) – if possible. A complete foot workout would probably take the beginner almost 1 hour, however, and sparing this amount of time is not easy.

The foot relaxation session (p.24)
The wonderfully relaxing effects of this session are alluded to throughout this book. Work through all the exercises on the right foot first, then treat the left foot, to induce a state of sublime torpor. When using individual exercises inbetween work on specific reflexes, always relax both feet.The more relaxed the receiver, the more effective the treatment.

The complete foot workout (p.26)
When offering the complete workout, treat the whole of the right foot before going on to the left. A recommended order of treatment is given opposite. Match the thumb to the foot on which you are working: use the right thumb to work the right foot, from the inside to the outside edge, supporting it with the left hand. Arrows on the drawings show only one working direction, but it is important always to work back over the same area in the opposite direction, changing your support and working hands, in order to contact the maximum number of reflexes.

As a general rule, work over individual reflexes 2 or 3 times, in each direction. If any reflexes are particularly sensitive, gently work over them again.

If time is of the essence, just work the principal reflexes indicated for specific ailments. Some of these may be covered in a matter of seconds – so always start with the general foot relaxation session and intersperse the treatment of specific reflexes with one or two relaxing exercises. Choose these intuitively, or offer the ones the receiver enjoys most.

When working on particular reflexes, treat the right foot first, then the left, as you go along. You are reminded of this at the end of each set of instructions. "Repeat on the left foot" naturally means changing the support hand and the working thumb

The complete hand workout (p.32)
Throughout this book readers are directed to the appropriate pages of the complete hand workout (pp. 32-37) for guidance on how to treat their own hands. This self-help therapy can be utilized anywhere at any time as a back up to treating the feet in the case of particular ailments or as an on-the-spot treatment to reduce tension and anxiety.

Cautionary notes
Seek professional advice from a doctor or qualified reflexologist before treating someone with diabetes, thrombosis, or phlebitis, or cancer patients who are undergoing conventional treatments.

Do not treat women in the first 14 weeks of pregnancy, particularly if they have a history of miscarriage.

Do not treat people in the acute stage of an infectious illness.

Do not attempt to diagnose problems according to sensitivities.

Working order: right foot

Start with diaphragm relaxation exercise
1 Work the lung/breast (sole and top of foot)
Metatarsal kneading exercise
2 Work the sinuses
3 Work the eye and ear
4 Work the neck, thyroid, and throat
5 Work the coccyx
6 Work the hip/pelvis
7 Work the spine
8 Work the brain
9 Work the face
10 Work the shoulder
11 Work the knee/elbow
12 Work the sciatic nerve
Side to side relaxation exercise
13R Work the liver and gallbladder
14R Work the ileocecal valve
15R Work the ascending, transverse colon,
and small intestine
Ankle freeing exercise
16 Work the bladder and ureter
17 Work the kidney
Under and overgrip relaxation
18 Work the uterus/prostate
19 Work the ovary/testis
20 Work the fallopian tube/vas deferens
Foot moulding and ribcage
relaxation exercises
Note any sensitive areas
'R' indicates reflexes found on right foot only.

Working order: left foot

Start with the diaphragm relaxation exercise
1 Work the lung/breast (sole and top of foot)
1A* Work the heart
Metatarsal kneading exercise
2 Work the sinuses
3 Work the eye and ear
4 Work the neck, thyroid and throat
5 Work the coccyx
6 Work the hip/pelvis
7 Work the spine
8 Work the brain
9 Work the face
10 Work the shoulder
11 Work the knee/elbow
12 Work the sciatic nerve
Side to side relaxation exercise
13L Work the stomach and pancreas
14L Work the spleen
15L Work the transverse, descending,
sigmoid colon, and small intestine
Ankle freeing exercise
16 Work the bladder and ureter
17 Work the kidney
17 Under- and overgrip relaxation
18 Work the uterus/prostate
19 Work the ovary/testis
20 Work the fallopian tube/vas deferens
Foot moulding and ribcage
relaxation exercises

Note any sensitive areas. Return to the right
foot and work 2 or 3 times over the sensitive
areas on that foot. Then do the same on the left
foot. The heart reflex 1A* is only on the left foot.
'L' indicates other reflexes only found on the left
foot. Working instructions are on p. 31.

Frequency of treatment

In acute cases, treat daily if possible
but at least 2 or 3 times a week.
When discomfort is reduced, once
weekly is enough. In chronic cases,
treat once or twice weekly until
improvement is noted. Then treat
once every 2 weeks, if improvement
is maintained, eventually reducing
to once monthly for a few months.

The foot relaxation session

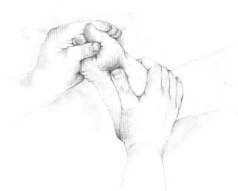

1 Relaxing the diaphragm
Start on the right foot, placing your left thumb beneath the toes, as shown. Work your right thumb across the diaphragm line, from the inside to the outside edge of the foot. While you are doing this, rock the toes back and forth across your left thumb. Edge the right thumb along each time you bend the toes over. (Repeat on the left foot.)

2 Side to side rocking
Support the right foot between the palms of the hands. Then gently but rapidly rock the foot from side to side between the hands. The motion should produce a distinctive flapping sound. (Repeat on the left foot.)

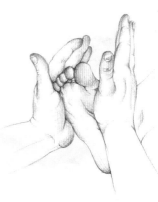

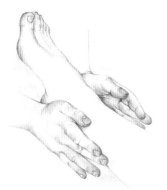

3 Freeing the ankle
Begin with the right foot. Support the ankle bones with the pads of your thumbs and rock the foot gently but rapidly from side to side, keeping your wrists loose. (Repeat on the left foot.)

4 Kneading the metatarsals
Push your right fist into the sole of the right foot, and the left hand over the top of the foot. Then, as if you were kneading dough, press the fist into the sole, while squeezing the top of the foot with the left hand. Start off slowly, and try to set up a gentle rhythm. (Repeat on the left foot.)

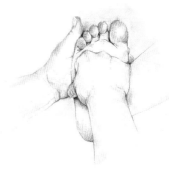

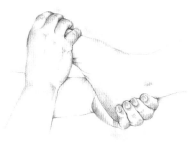

5 Circling with undergrip
Support the right heel in the palm of the left hand, with the thumb on the outside edge. Lightly hold the top of the foot with your right hand and turn the foot inward, making clockwise circling movements. (Repeat on the left foot.)

6 Circling with overgrip
Apply pressure with your left hand over the top of the right ankle. With your right hand, turn the foot inward, making light circling movements. This is an excellent exercise for reducing swollen ankles. (Repeat on the left foot.)

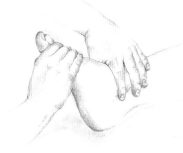

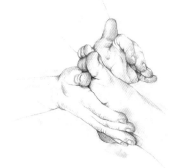

7 Moulding the foot
Cradle the right foot between your hands, supporting it on the outside edge. Now work across the top and sole of the foot, rotating the hands, like the wheels of a train. (Repeat on the left foot.)

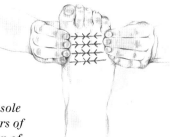

8 Relaxing the ribcage
Begin on the right foot, pressing into the sole with both thumbs and work all the fingers of each hand toward each other over the top of the foot. (Repeat on the left foot.)

The complete workout: right foot

1 Work the lungs and breast

First work the sole of the right foot, supporting it as shown. With your right thumb, work up each area from the diaphragm line to the base of each toe. Then work down the grooves on top of the foot with your index finger. Open them up by making a fist with your left hand and pushing into the sole.

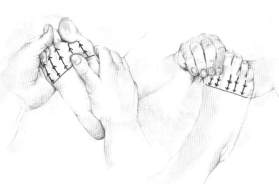

2 Work the sinuses

Support the top of the right foot with your left hand. Use your right thumb to work up all the toes, starting at the base of the big toe. When you reach the little toe, change hands and work back in the opposite direction.

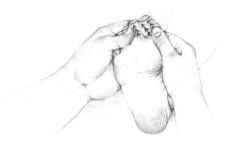

3 Work the eyes and ears

Support the right foot with your left hand. To contact the eye reflex, place your right thumb under the first bend of the second toe, and make small clockwise rotations.

   Work the ear reflex, under the first bend of the third toe, in exactly the same way.

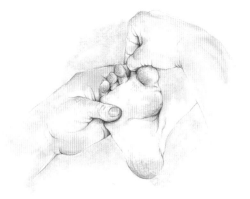

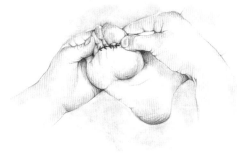

4 Work the neck, thyroid, and throat

Support the right foot with your left hand. Use your right thumb to work across the line where the first 3 toes join the foot. (For throat problems, concentrate mainly on the base of the big toe.) Then work across the base of the 3 toes on the top of the foot with the right index finger (see p. 106).

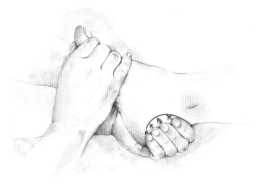

5 Work the coccyx

Work on the important spine reflex usually begins with the coccyx. With your right hand, hold the top of the right foot away from the body. With all 4 fingers of the left hand, make small forward creeping movements, starting on the back edge of the heel and stopping at the point shown in the drawing.

6 Work the hip and pelvis

Use your left hand to support the top of the right foot, tilting it away from the body. Use all 4 fingers of your right hand to creep around the outside edge of the heel, covering the area shown in the drawing.

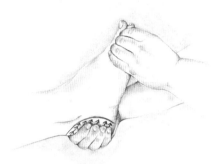

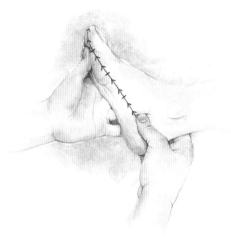

7 Work the spine

The spine reflex points follow the line of the inside edge of the foot; they are not on the sole. With your left hand, hold the right foot away from the body, and use your right thumb to creep, "pincushion" fashion, along the line shown up to the top of the big toe.

8 Work the brain

Support the top of the right foot with your left hand. With your right thumb, apply pressure to the top of the big toe. Hold to a count of 3 and release. Do this 4 or 5 times. Treat the tops of the second and third toes in the same way.

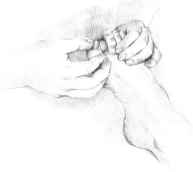

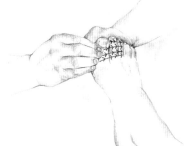

9 Work the face

Push your left fist behind the toes on the right foot. This acts as a support while you work out the area below the toe nails on the first 3 toes. With your right index finger, start just below the nail and work down to the base on each toe.

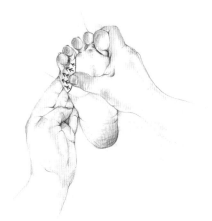

10 Work the shoulder

Support the right foot with your left hand. Use your right thumb to work the segment of the foot shown beneath the fourth and fifth toes, starting at the top.

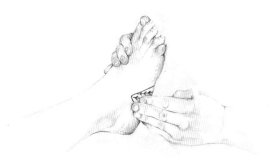

11 Work the knee and elbow

Use your right hand to support the right foot. With your left index finger, work in all directions over the triangular area on the side of the foot. (The apex of the triangle aligns with the bony protuberance on the side of the foot.)

12 Work the sciatic nerve

With your right hand, support the right foot. Place your left index finger just behind the ankle bone, and work in a line up the leg for about 10cm (4in).

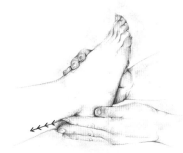

13 R Work the liver and gallbladder

Support the top of the right foot with your left hand and use your right thumb to work from the inside to the outside edge in the direction shown. When your reach the outside edge, change hands and work back in the opposite direction.

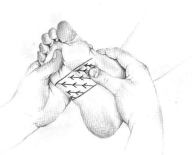

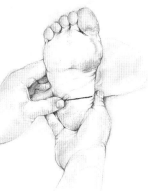

14 R Work the ileocecal valve

This reflex is only on the right foot. Work it with a "hooking out" technique. Supporting the heel with your right hand, use your left thumb to press down on the outside edge of the pelvic line. Then, still maintaining the pressure, pull the thumb back toward you, releasing pressure (but not contact) at the end of the movement. Do this 3 times.

15 R Work the ascending, transverse colon, and small intestine

Support the heel with your left hand. Use your right thumb to work across the area between the waist and the pelvic line in the direction shown. Then change hands and work back in the opposite direction.

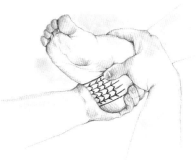

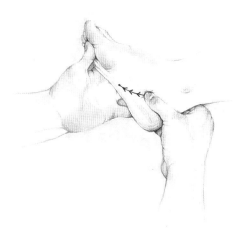

16 Work the bladder and ureter

Support the right foot with your left hand. With your right thumb, work over the soft, puffy area on the inside edge of the foot. Then work up the foot with small creeping movements, along the ureter reflex, as indicated, up to the kidney. Make sure you work on the inside edge of the ligament line. Working directly on it causes extreme discomfort.

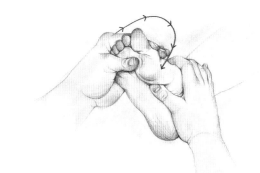

17 Work the kidneys

The kidney reflex is just below the diaphragm line, to the left of the ligament line. In most people it is a sensitive point and the following way of working is likely to cause least discomfort.

Support the right foot with your left hand. Press your right thumb into the kidney reflex point and maintain the pressure while you gently rotate the foot around the thumb, using your left hand.

18 Work the uterus/prostate

Support the right foot with your left hand. Use your right index finger to work the area indicated from the edge of the heel up to the ankle bone. Repeat on the left foot.

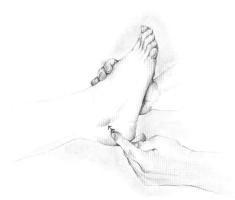

19 Work the ovaries/testes

Hold the right foot with your right hand, tilting the foot outward to relax the muscles and ligaments in the ankles. Use your left index finger to work in a straight line from the base of the heel up to the ankle bone.

20 Work the fallopian tube/vas deferens

Use both hands for each foot. First press the thumbs into the sole of the foot to bring the top into relief. Then, starting as low as possible on the sides, work the first 2 fingers of each hand across the foot in front of the ankle bone.

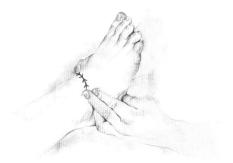

Working reflexes located only on the left foot

1A* Work the heart (after the lungs)

Support the top of the left foot with your right hand and use your left thumb to work the area shown, starting at the base of the big toe and working across to the third toe. Never overwork this area (3 times maximum) and give the diaphragm relaxation exercise (p. 24) after treating it.

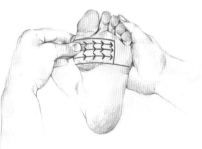

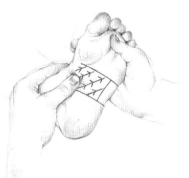

13L Work the stomach and pancreas

Support the left foot with your right hand and use your left thumb to work the area indicated. When you reach the outside limit of the area, change hands and work back in the opposite direction.

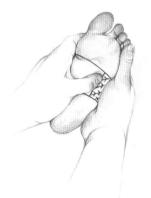

14L Work the spleen

Supporting the left foot with the right hand, use your left thumb to work the oblong area indicated on the outside edge of the foot between the diaphragm line and the waist line.

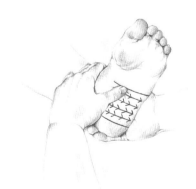

15L Work the transverse, descending, sigmoid colon, and the small intestine

With your right hand, support the heel of the left foot. Use your left thumb to work across the foot, from the inside to the outside edge, from the waist line to below the pelvic line. Change hands and work back over the area in the opposite direction.

The complete hand workout

Hand reflexology is an important self-help strategy. Use it as a back up to work on the feet in the case of common ailments (Chapter Four) or stress-related conditions (Chapter Five). In both chapters readers are directed to the appropriate pages of the complete hand workout. As with the feet, regular treatments help to boost your general vitality, so make the workout a pleasurable routine (see p. 21). Treat all the reflexes on the right hand first, then the left.

A knowledge of the hand reflexes is always useful for the reflexologist who will almost inevitably encounter situations where it is not possible to treat the feet because of localized infection or injury.

1 Work the lung and breast
First work the palm of the right hand. With your left thumb, work across the area between the diaphragm line and the point where the fingers start.

Work on the palm of the hand focuses mainly on the lung area. (Repeat on the left hand.)

2 Work the breast and lung
Now work the top of the hand. Place your left index finger on the point where the finger joins the hand and work down the groove for about 2.5cm (1in).

Working the top of the hand focuses mainly on the breast area.

(Repeat on the left hand. Then work the heart reflex ,see p. 37).

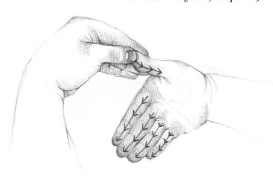

3 Work the sinuses
Work the right hand first, using your left thumb to work the reflex points down the length of the thumb and all the fingers. When working your own hand, it is easier to do this if you start at the tips of thumb and fingers. If working on someone else, work up the fingers from the base. (Repeat on the left hand.)

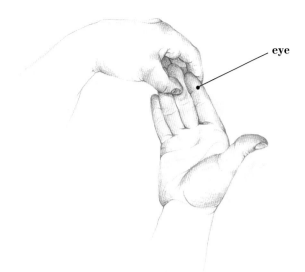

eye

4 Work the eye and ear

To work the eye, use your left thumb to make small clockwise rotating movements over the reflex on the first bend of the right index finger.

To work the ear, use the same technique on the reflex point on the first joint of the middle finger. (Repeat on the left hand.)

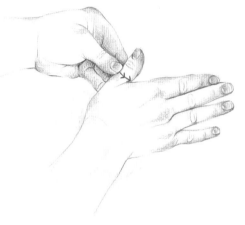

5 Work the neck, thyroid, and throat

With your left thumb, work the thyroid reflexes which form a ring around the base of the thumb. At the same time you are contacting the throat reflexes. By working the bases of the next 2 fingers, you relieve neck and shoulder tension. (Repeat on the left hand.)

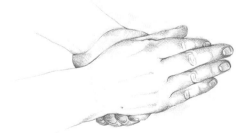

6 Work the coccyx, hip, and pelvis

Use the 4 fingers of your left hand to apply pressure to the outside edge of your right hand. Start on the lower edge, to contact the coccyx, then edge up the side to contact the reflexes for the hip and pelvis on the top of the hand. (Repeat on the left hand.)

The complete hand workout 33

7 Work the spine

*Use your left thumb to work along the
line indicated on the right palm in order
to contact the reflex points for the spine.*
*(Repeat, following the corresponding
line, on the left hand.)*

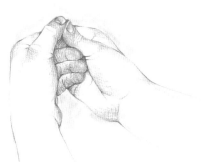

8 Work the brain

*Use your left thumb to work the top of the
right thumb. Apply pressure, hold it for 5
seconds, and then release. Do this 3 times.
(Repeat on the left hand.)*

9 Work the face and teeth

*Use your left thumb to work across the
right thumb, starting below the nail,
and following the lines indicated.
Then work the same area on the index
and middle fingers. (Repeat on the left
hand.)*

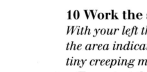

10 Work the shoulder

*With your left thumb, apply pressure to
the area indicated, edging forward with
tiny creeping movements..*
*To contact the reflex points for the left
shoulder, repeat on the left hand. For
balance, it is always best to work the
reflexes on both hands.*

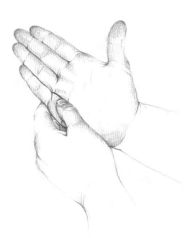

11 Work the knee and elbow

With your left index and middle fingers, work the triangular area on the outside edge of the right hand. (Repeat on the left hand.)

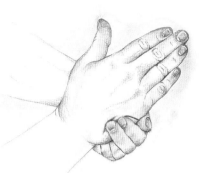

12 R Work the liver and gallbladder

The reflexes for these are only on the right hand. Use your left thumb to work the area shown on the right palm.

(On the left palm, work the reflexes for the stomach, pancreas, and spleen, see 12 L, p. 37.)

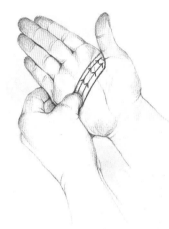

13 Work the intestines

Use your left thumb to work the area indicated on the palm of the right hand. This contacts the ascending, transverse colon, and small intestine.

(Work the same area on the left hand to contact the transverse, descending, sigmoid colon.)

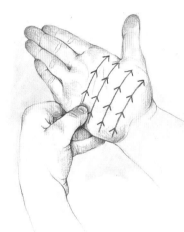

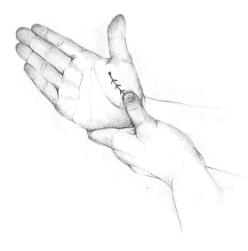

14 Work the bladder and ureter

Apply pressure with your left thumb to the fleshy pad of the right palm, just below the thumb. This contacts the bladder reflex. Now continue edging on up the line indicated, toward the base of the index finger, where you contact the ureter. (Repeat on the left hand.)

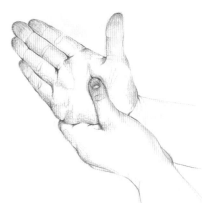

15 Work the kidneys

With the left thumb, work on from the end of the ureter line (see step 16) to the kidney reflex which is near the point where the thumb joins the hand. Work over this area in all directions. (Repeat on the left hand.)

16 Work the uterus/prostate

With your left thumb, work the reflex point that is located just below the thumb of the right hand. This reflex is linked by the fallopian tube/vas deferens "bracelet" with the ovary/testis reflex. (Repeat on the left hand.)

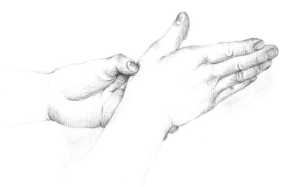

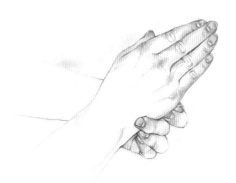

17 Work the ovary/testis (and groin lymph)

Use the middle finger of your left hand to contact and work the reflex points on the outside edge of the hand, just in front of the wrist bone. This area is on the "bracelet" formed around the wrist by the fallopian tube/vas deferens reflexes. Repeat on the left hand.

18 Work the fallopian tube/vas deferens

Use either the left thumb or the forefinger to work these reflexes, which encircle the wrist, like a bracelet. Repeat on the left hand.

Working reflexes found only on the left hand

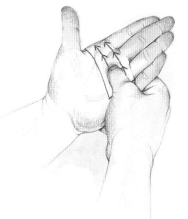

Work the heart

On the left hand, work this reflex after you have worked the lung and chest area. Use your right thumb to work over the area indicated on the left palm. As on the feet, do not overwork this reflex. Going over it 2 or 3 times is sufficient.

12 L Work the stomach, pancreas, spleen, and solar plexus

With your right thumb, work over the area indicated on the left palm. Because the working area on the hand is so much smaller than that on the foot, it is easy to treat the spleen every time you treat the intestines. Work on this area in any odd moment, since working the spleen helps boost immunity.

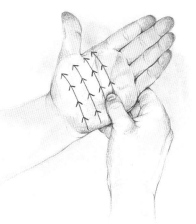

Chapter Two

Living Life to the Full

Living life to the full means caring for yourself on every level, ensuring that your physical, mental, and spiritual needs are nourished and in a state of dynamic harmony.

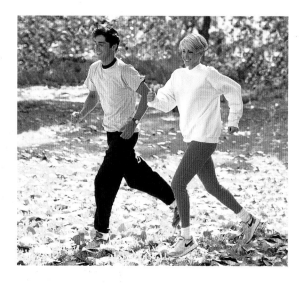

***Pleasure and persistence** are key ingredients of a successful exercise programme. Devise one that is varied and appropriate for your age and general level of health.*

Regular exercise keeps you healthy, strong, and supple, while building up protection against heart disease, improving circulation, keeping weight down, and reducing stress.

Throughout this book "support strategies" suggest ways in which you can enhance or accelerate the holistic healing process by backing up reflexology with other so-called "alternative" therapies or treatments. As well as a number of folk remedies, these include relaxation, meditation, aromatherapy, and herbalism. There are numerous excellent publications and practical courses you can turn to if you wish to explore any of the support strategies in depth. This chapter proposes a brief introduction to those most frequently recommended. None is intended to replace conventional medical advice or treatment.

Before rushing off to enroll in a yoga class, however, review certain basic aspects of your everyday living. It is unrealistic to expect results from any form of treatment if you persist in eating all the wrong foods, in smoking, or in drinking too much, while remaining resolutely slumped in an armchair. Eating a healthy diet and taking brisk regular exercise are, therefore, essential first steps in increasing your general level of vitality.

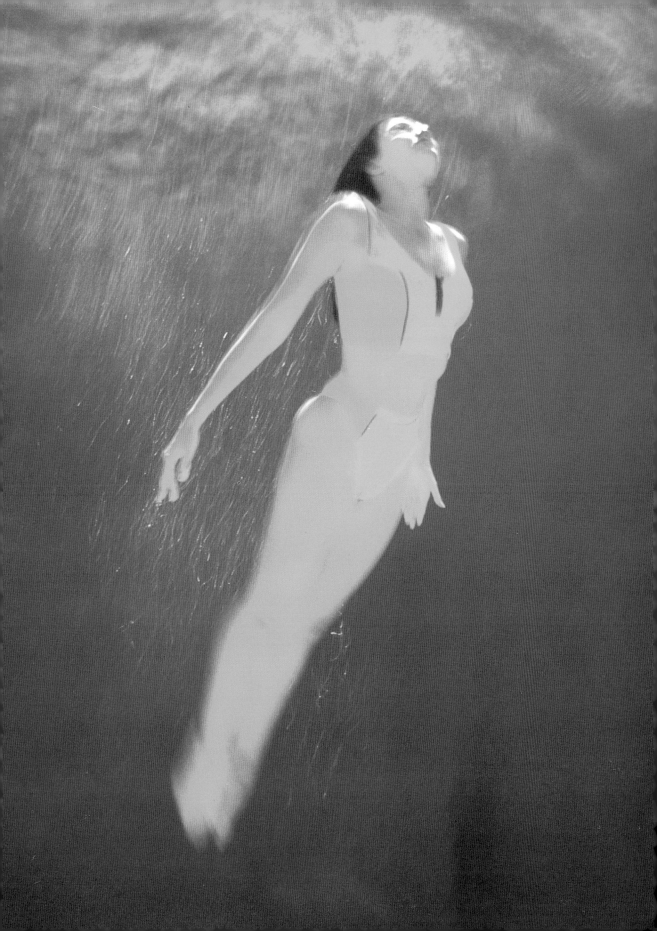

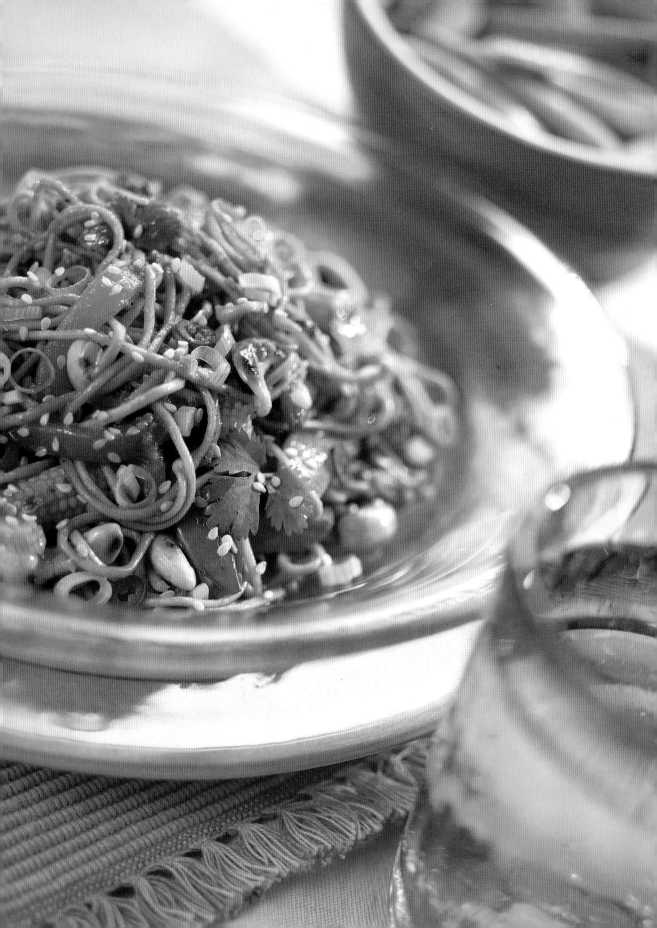

You *are* what you eat!

Feeling energetic, vibrant, and well is the natural state of any healthy being. And in order to maintain, or achieve, this state of wellbeing, a healthy, balanced diet is essential. As an adult you are responsible for your own diet; as a parent, you are also responsible for that of your children – and good eating habits are established in infancy.

In order to function well, to repair, and regenerate, the body needs good fuel, provided in as natural a state as possible. Fresh fruits and vegetables (eaten raw as often as possible), grains, pulses, rice, and wholemeal bread are some of the building blocks of good health. Hamburgers, cola drinks (with a high caffeine content), chocolate, chips, and highly processed foods are not. Sugars, caffeine, and food preservatives lack trace nutrients, and contribute nothing to the body, while placing a number of strains on its systems.

The joy of physical fitness

The importance of regular exercise, whatever your age, cannot be overstressed. Essential for muscle tone and function, including the muscle of the heart, it also stimulates the circulatory, digestive, and respiratory systems. Choose a form of exercise that you enjoy and that you are likely to be able to pursue on a regular basis. Ideally, try to devise a 3-point programme, which includes aerobic, stretching, and relaxing exercises. Such a combination of exercises is highly effective in treating a variety of disorders, from obesity and addictions to anxiety and depression.

If you are not in the habit of exercising, do not overdo it to begin with. If you are seriously overweight, take medical advice before even starting on an exercise programme. If you decide to jog or run, for

First steps to healthy eating

A balanced diet includes sources of carbohydrate, fats, protein, vitamins, and minerals. If you suspect that your family's diet needs attention or rebalancing, consider taking the following actions:

Eat at least 5 portions of fresh fruit and vegetables daily. Steam or stir-fry vegetables to preserve vitamin and mineral content.

◆

Eat wholemeal bread instead of white.

◆

Eat low-fat chicken or game instead of fatty meats such as pork. Increase your fatty fish intake.

◆

Replace one or two meat meals each week with dishes made from lentils, pulses, wholewheat pasta, rice, seeds, or nuts.

◆

Drink 1-2 litres (2-4 pints) of water a day.

◆

Reduce your overall intake of animal products (dairy and meat).

◆

Reduce your intake of salt and caffeine (tea, coffee, cola drinks). Avoid sugars.

◆

Do not drink more than 1-2 units of alcohol per day.

◆

Use mono-unsaturated oil (cold pressed olive oil) or polyunsaturated oils (sesame, soya, sunflower), or non-hydrogenated margarines for cooking.

aerobic exercise, always do so on a soft surface, such as grass; the impact of feet on hard pavements sends shock waves to the hips that would shatter them if they were made of steel, and long-term pavement joggers often need hip replacements in later life. If you are not up to jogging, a daily brisk walk, for about half an hour, is equally beneficial. Yoga asanas (postures) are excellent for toning and stretching all the muscles of the body. After working your muscles hard, allow them gently to relax, following the technique outlined below.

The revitalizing breath
Clarity of mind and increased vitality are the positive spinoffs of breathing to your full capacity. In addition, breathing "properly" helps to reduce the effects of respiratory disorders, as well as to alleviate anxiety, depression, and fatigue.

Shaking off a lifetime's habit of shallow breathing requires application and understanding of the physical mechanisms of breathing. Begin by learning some simple exercises that will encourage diaphragm breathing. To get used to this, you first have to become familiar with the "feel" of breathing deeply into the abdomen.

Lie flat on the floor with a pillow under your head and another under your knees. If you cannot lie on the floor, sit on a chair with a straight back. Relax and breathe normally. Now place your hands, with fingertips touching, on your navel area, just below the ribs. Breathe in deeply through the nose, directing the breath to this area. You should feel your fingers part as the abdomen rises. As you breathe out, contract the abdominal muscles to expel as much air as possible. Repeat this for 6 breaths.

Once you are aware of the way in which the upper ribs, chest, and abdomen expand

as you breathe in and contract as you breathe out, you can repeat this deep breathing at any time during the day.

In order for correct breathing to become habitual, you need training. This would form part of most yoga classes, as well, of course, of tai chi or chi kung (energy work). In the meantime, you can begin your chosen relaxation technique with a few deep breaths into the abdomen, consciously letting go any tensions on the out breath.

Renewal through relaxation
An important part of achieving mental and physical wellbeing is caring, really caring, for yourself. And this includes giving yourself a break on a regular basis – preferably every day. If you are able to, reserve a room in the house to which you can retreat and where you can, if you wish, listen to relaxing music while going through a simple total body relaxation exercise. If you are feeling particularly fraught at any time, drop everything and do the exercise there and then. It will break the spiral of tension, and allow you to resume your activities in a calmer, controlled state.

Lie flat on the floor, arms by your side, and palms upward. Let your feet fall outward at the ankles. (Have a thin pillow or a paperback book under your head for support, if you wish.)

Take half a dozen breaths deep into the abdomen. Then continue to breathe gently and naturally.

Starting with the little toe on the left foot, direct your attention to every part of your body, naming that part in your mind, as you do so. Do no more than that. Do not tense the part, just name it, then move on to the next. Do not rush.

Begin with the toes: left little toe, etc. Ball of left foot, left instep, left heel, left ankle,

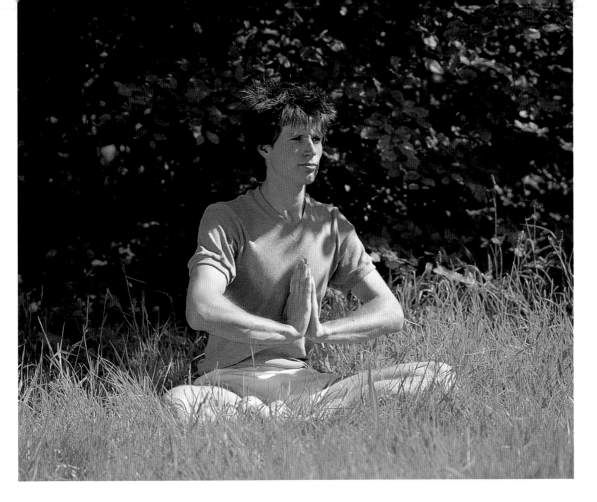

left calf, back of left knee, left thigh, left buttock, left waist, left side, left shoulder blade, left shoulder, top of left arm, left elbow, lower left arm, left wrist, left palm, left little finger, etc. Repeat this process on the right side of the body. Then direct your attention to the centre of the body, working up the spinal vertebrae to the neck. All the time, just name the parts. By the time you have gone through all of them, you will be deeply relaxed. Use this technique to help you drop off to sleep at night, if necessary.

Yoga for mind-body harmony

The oldest system of self-development in the world, yoga originated in India thousands of years ago. The asanas or postures that are the essential feature of hatha yoga, the branch most commonly pursued in the West,

*A **state of inner peace**, in which the mind is stilled yet dynamic and alert, may arise through regular yoga practice. This state may long elude you, but other benefits of yoga are felt right from the start, and can be enjoyed at any age.*

exercise "every muscle, nerve, and gland in the body" according to the world authority and leading yoga teacher, B.K.S. Iyengar.

Different asanas stretch and tone muscles, keep the spine and joints supple, and massage internal organs. Special breathing techniques (for which a teacher is essential) further increase the amounts of oxygen in the bloodstream and, like the asanas, encourage the flow of prana (the life force).

Yoga means "union" – specifically the union of the spirit with the Absolute, or with God. It is thus concerned not only with the

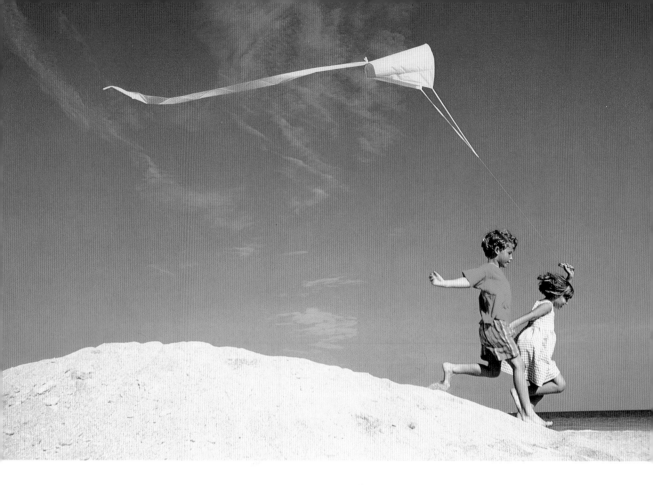

Just being in the moment, *in the way that children are, is the goal of many adults. The principles of meditation may suggest ways of preventing invasive thoughts about the past or future marring your enjoyment of the present.*

physical being, but with the totality of the individual. Whether you practise meditation along with yoga, or whether you consider the asanas themselves as a form of meditation, over a period of time you will observe that regular practice leads to subtle inner changes, perhaps reflecting a sense of greater harmony between your self and the outside world.

You can practise yoga at any age. If you are an absolute beginner, however, take lessons from an experienced teacher. Learn at your own pace. Yoga is totally uncompetitive, and you do not need to force yourself. You will

find, however, that the real benefits derive from practising at home what you have learned in your class.

Try to set aside a regular time each day, whether first thing in the morning or last thing at night, when you can devote at least a quarter of an hour to yoga.

Meditation and inner serenity

The regular practice of meditation, stilling the mind and emptying it of circling, nagging thoughts, leads eventually to an awareness of an Inner Self – a source of strength, wisdom, and guidance.

Achieving this stillness, however, letting go unwanted thoughts, is no easy matter. The beginner, therefore, is advised first to master concentration.

Set aside 10 minutes twice a day – perhaps first thing in the morning, then later in the evening (but leave 2 hours after a meal). Choose a quiet spot where you will be comfortable, warm, and undisturbed. Take the telephone off the hook.

Sit or kneel on the floor or sit on an upright chair (not one that you will drop off to sleep in). Make sure that you are comfortable since physical discomfort will distract you. Feel the weight of your body on the chair or floor.

Check every part of the body for tension, and gently let it go. Relax the jaw and let the eyes sink softly back into their sockets.

Do not attempt to banish thoughts from your mind. Rather, just observe them, as you might passersby in the street. Watch them come, and go.

Then direct your attention to the breath, feeling the passage of cool air as it enters your nostrils. Follow it in your mind as it passes down your windpipe into the lungs. Then, as you breathe out, be aware that it is slightly warmer as it is expelled through your nostrils.

Counting the breath is a tried and tested technique. Do this on an exhalation, in cycles of 4 breaths for about 5 minutes. If you are distracted, direct your attention to the sensation of the breath entering and leaving the body, then begin counting again.

Alternatively, concentrate on a lighted candle or a single flower set before you in a simple container. The silent internal repetition of a mantra (a word or phrase that has special meaning for you) is a technique favoured by many.

Visualization is another: simply picture in your mind's eye a place where you always feel at peace, or picture a gently flowing stream, a flowery meadow in the sun, whatever images conjure feelings of serenity. If visualization works for you, it would be interesting to try offering a "guided visualization" along with your reflexology treatment. As you work their feet, gently talk the receiver through a walk in the country or along a beach.

The tonic, uplifting effects of regular meditation benefit both the mental and physical body. Blood pressure is lowered, the immune system is improved, the digestive system works more efficiently, and the heart beat slows to a restful pace. Particularly effective in stress-related conditions, regular meditation is superior to all the sleeping pills and tranquillizers so abundantly prescribed in the western world today. Nonetheless, it is not recommended for everyone and it may not suit you if you are deeply depressed (see below).

Active meditation
If you find it difficult to remain still to meditate, or if it makes you feel anxious, you can make more physical activities, such as the yoga asanas, the slow and expressive movements of tai chi or the meditative postures of chi kung, or even simply walking or running, your own preferred form of active meditation.

Meditation & introspection

If you are depressed and prone to introspection, it is not advisable to take up meditation. Opt, rather, for a more physical form of meditative exercise, such as yoga. And in yoga, concentrate on the standing poses that encourage opening upward and outward, rather than the forward bending poses that turn you in on yourself.

Healing fragrances: aromatherapy

Essential oils, or essences, obtained by distilling the leaves, flowers, stems, or bark of aromatic plants and trees, have a number of healing properties. With certain caveats, outlined below, most essential oils can safely be used to treat all members of the family. Some have anti-inflammatory properties, others (notably tea tree oil) are valuable antiseptics. Some have a stimulating, others a calming effect. Choose the ones most suited to your needs and which appeal to you as fragrances.

Added to a base or carrier oil for massage, they penetrate the skin, helping to heal muscles and internal organs. Inhaled through the nose, some seem to activate deep areas of the brain and act on the nervous system, to reduce anxiety. Never inhale neat oil straight from the bottle (particularly if you are asthmatic, it could trigger an attack). Use a few drops in your bath, or in a vaporizer to fill your room with healing fragrance.

Always use the best quality essential oil, adding 2 drops to 5ml (a teaspoon) of carrier or base oil. Store the oil in a tightly stoppered dark glass bottle and keep it in a cool place. You may blend oils according to your needs and preference. For the carrier oil, choose a cold-pressed virgin vegetable oil, such as almond, walnut, sunflower, or grapeseed oil.

Massage

Either use the oil for a full-body massage or use it to treat specific problem areas. When massaging, always work toward the heart, and on the abdomen work clockwise in circles.

Baths

First close the bathroom window and door, to contain the fragrance. Then add 7 or 8 drops of neat oil to the tub just before you get in, swooshing it around to disperse it in the water. Relax for 10 minutes or so in the bath, enjoying the effects of the oil on the skin and in the air.

Inhalations

For catarrh, blocked nose, or sore throat, float 2-3 drops of an appropriate oil on the surface of about half a litre (a pint) of

Use oils with caution

Never take oils by mouth, except under medical supervision.

◆

Never use neat oils on the skin. If you have a skin allergy, seek professional advice before using them.

◆

Halve the quantities for children under 13 years of age. Quarter them for under 13s.

◆

Pregnant women should only accept aromatherapy from a qualified practitioner.

◆

If you suffer from an allergy or asthma, never inhale oils neat direct from the bottle.

◆

Never use oil burners in a bedroom overnight, or in a child's room at any time. Oils are flammable. Keep them away from naked flames.

◆

If a child swallows an oil, seek medical advice at once. This is an emergency.

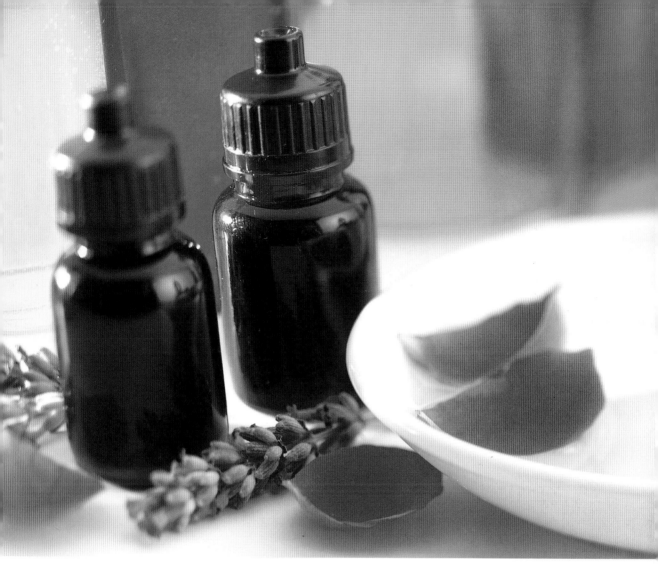

steaming water. Drape a towel over your head, close your eyes and breathe in the steam for 2-3 minutes. Do not do this if you suffer from asthma or an allergy.

Vaporizers
Use an oil burner with a candle, as long as it is continually supervised. If you want to enjoy aromatherapy while you sleep, it is safer to use an electric vaporizer. Use 5 or 6 drops of oil to about 15ml (3 teaspoons) of water for an oil burner. Follow the instructions supplied with electric vaporizers.

Aromatherapy oils are expensive, since a sea of petals or leaves is needed to produce just a drop of essential oil. But the distilled oil is so powerful that a little goes a long way.

Massage for a sense of wholeness
Like reflexology, massage is a way of communicating loving care and concern, without words. The healing power of touch is harnessed to soothe and relax muscles knotted with tension or to encourage mental strains to dissipate. At the same time, in a full-body massage, both giver and receiver enter into a state of communion, likened by

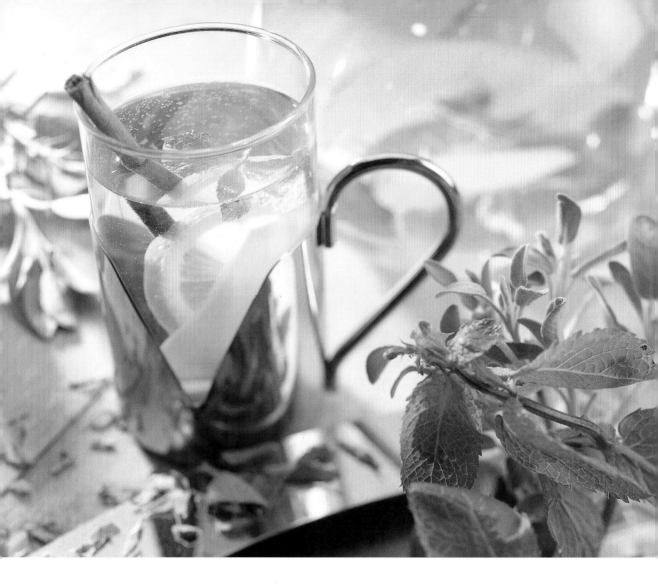

Fresh or dried herbs *can be used to make healing teas that are most potent when freshly brewed. Flavour them with honey, lemon, or a culinary herb, such as mint, and start taking them at the onset of symptoms.*

some to a meditation, in which they are both stilled and energized at the same time.

As well as the full-body massage, which may, incidentally, unlock deep-seated emotions which have long lain unexpressed (and you should be aware of this possibility), massage can be used in addition to reflexology for on the spot relief from tension, particularly in the neck area.

Babies love and thrive on it, and both parents can become involved in a regular simple routine that enhances and deepens the natural bonding process (see p. 61). Old people also respond well, particularly if after the loss of a partner they have been deprived of regular physical contact with others.

You can massage intuitively or learn various gliding, kneading, stroking, circling, and stretching techniques that are appropriate on particular areas of the body. Most important, is that you are "present" or "centred" throughout the session, and for this you may wish to prepare yourself mentally in advance.

For the massage, choose a quiet, warm, comfortable, pleasant setting where you are not likely to be interrupted. If necessary, in cold weather supply supplementary heating. Prepare everything in advance: the base oil (a good almond oil will do) and any aromatherapy essences that you are going to use. You can give the massage on the floor, or if it is more comfortable for you, on a table. Pad the surface with a couple of blankets, covered with towels. But do not be tempted to use a mattress since it is not resilient enough. Have your oils, warmed if necessary, close at hand where they cannot be knocked over. If necessary, cover the part of the body that you are not working on with a soft, warm towel. Have a large warm towel ready as covering at the end of the session.

If the person you are working on is not comfortable lying down, you can give a back massage while they sit in an ordinary dining chair. This is all the more effective if they can sit astride the chair. Cover the back of the chair with a pillow for comfort. You may like to listen to pleasant, relaxing music, but avoid chatting while you work. It is distracting and diminishes the impact of massage.

Natural healing with herbal remedies

The healing properties of plants and herbs have been recognized and used all over the world for thousands of years. Largely neglected, in western urban societies at any rate, over recent decades, herbs are now enjoying a resurgence of interest with more and more people growing them not only for culinary use but for medicinal purposes. Always seek the advice of a qualified medical herbalist before embarking on any prolonged use of a particular herb. In general, their short-term use is safe.

Use herbs as a tonic or as a sedative, to help prevent infection, to boost immunity, and to stimulate the circulatory system. While some can be bought ready packaged as teas, you can make your own infusions or decoctions, following the instructions below. One cup 3 times a day is the usual adult dose. Consult a qualified herbalist before giving herbal remedies to young children.

Healing Teas

Standard infusion
(using flowers, leaves, stems)

Use 28g (1oz) dried herb or 56g (2oz) fresh herb to 600ml (1 pint) water.

1 Warm the pot, and add the herbs.

2 Add boiling water and cover.

3 Infuse for 10 minutes.

4 Strain and drink.

In the case of chronic ailments, take 3 cups daily. In acute situations, take 1 or 2 cups every hour.

◆

Standard decoction
(using woody parts of plant)

Use the same quantities as for infusions, but use a little more water since decoctions need to boil and some will be lost through evaporation.

1 Crush or chop the bark, seeds, nuts, or root into small pieces.

2 Place in a pan (not aluminium) and cover with water.

3 Bring to the boil and simmer for 10-15 minutes.

4 Strain and drink.

Chapter Three

Healthy Babies
and Children

Use reflexology to stimulate your child's natural healing energy in times of crisis. Regular treatments help boost the immune system and prevent illness.

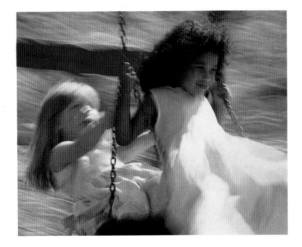

When the life force flows unimpeded *our zest for living is unbounded. Families who make reflexology part of their regular routine reap the benefits of this gentle, caring treatment in inner balance, harmony, and vitality.*

Most babies are not born fearful, timid, or tense. They enter the world untainted by the emotional wear and tear of the living process which, to a greater or lesser degree, eventually affects most people. So the life force in the newly born usually flows without restraint.

A head start for a healthy life
Babies are extremely sensitive to atmosphere, sound, temperature, and, of course, touch. Use reflexology from the word go, to give your child a head start in life. Brothers and sisters as well as parents can give gentle treatments to tiny feet, not only to help soothe and assuage the discomfort of colic or teething but to establish and nurture loving bonds with the new member of the family.

Children who are brought up with reflexology as part of their everyday family life and who receive, and give, treatments on a regular basis are likely to be more resistant to common ailments such as coughs, colds, and upset stomachs. More than this, the constant demonstration of

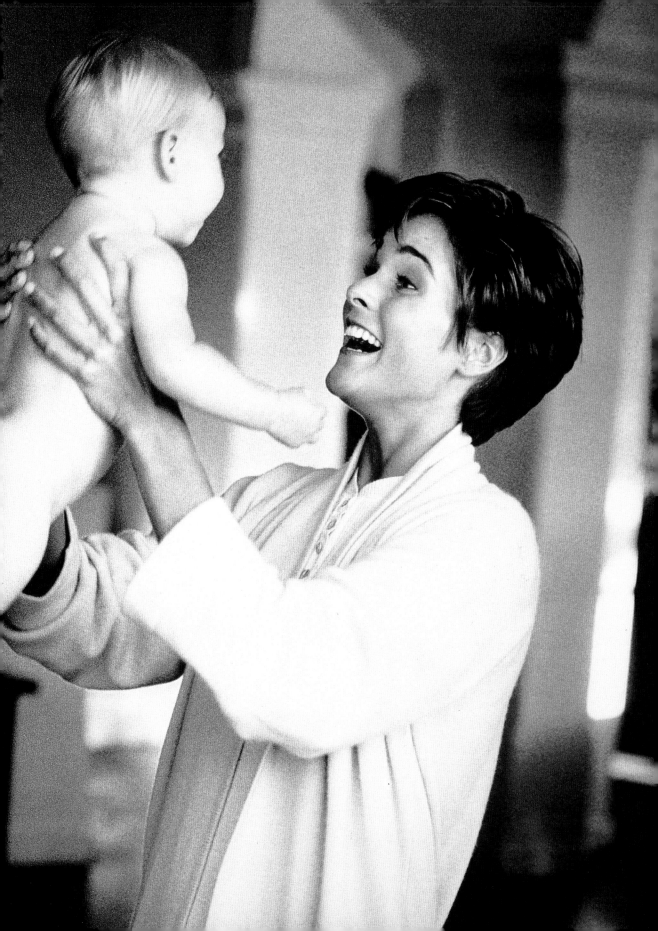

Causes for concern

Don't delay in seeking medical advice if it is difficult to rouse your baby from sleep or if he or she has any of the following symptoms:

◆

A temperature over 39ºC (102ºF) in a child under 3 months of age

◆

Fast, laboured breathing during which the chest pulls in

◆

Diarrhea or vomiting

◆

Fits or seizures

◆

Screaming with drawn-up legs and the stomach does not relax between screams

tender loving care from members of their family helps build their self-esteem and confidence as well as sensitivity toward the needs of others.

Clear channels for energy healing

Nothing is more agonizing for a new parent than to see a tiny baby in obvious distress – for no obvious reason. Though discomfiting, the cause is not often serious. For the most common causes of crying in the early weeks and months – digestive upsets and teething – reflexology is an effective and harmless treatment you can employ to give your baby (and yourself) some relief.

The very young respond particularly readily to reflexology. Not only is their life force extremely strong, their organic functioning is also sound. The impediments to healing found in many adults, whether due to the detrimental effects of long-term exposure to common environmental

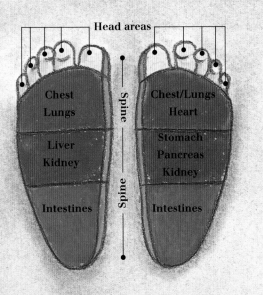

Head areas

Chest
Lungs

Liver
Kidney

Intestines

Spine

Chest/Lungs
Heart

Stomach
Pancreas
Kidney

Intestines

The foot maps: 0–3 year olds

Until the age of 3 the feet are roughly oval in form, since the arches have not yet developed. Although the shape gives few clues to the position of reflex points, the broad divisions indicated here are useful if you need to concentrate on particular areas. With such small feet, however, it is easy to cover the whole foot several times at every treatment.

To do this, start on the inside of the right foot and, with a tiny forward creeping movement of the thumb, gently work up from the base of the heel to the point where the toes join the foot. Work in this way across the foot to the outside edge, and repeat on the left foot. In this way you cover all the energy zones and treat most of the body systems (see pp. 54–55).

pollutants, to years of medication, inappropriate diet, or various forms of over-indulgence, are simply not present in a strong young body.

Cuddling, caressing, and stroking your baby are natural expressions of your joy in their being and an essential part of the bonding process. In some parts of the world, mothers make a full-body massage a part of the baby's daily routine (see p. 61). If at this early stage you can make work on the feet an accepted part of your times of loving physical contact, the baby will soon learn to love it.

A baby's foot is so small that it takes very little time to work over the entire sole with your thumb or finger. Use only the gentlest of pressure, since the area is sensitive and the foot not yet fully formed. Work on the feet for about 5 minutes. It is perfectly safe to repeat the routine every hour, if necessary, until the baby settles and sleeps.

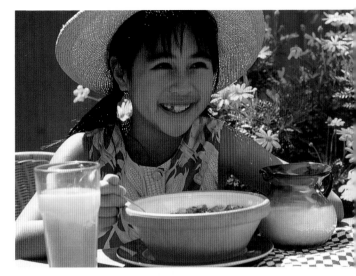

Radiant health and wellbeing reflect an inner state of harmony and balance. It is every parent's wish that their child should enjoy optimum health and vitality. A loving family, a healthy diet, and – yes! – regular reflexology treatments will help ensure that they do.

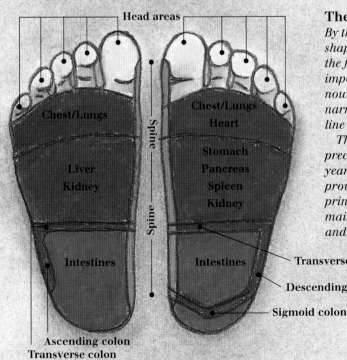

Head areas

Chest/Lungs
Spine
Chest/Lungs
Heart

Stomach
Pancreas
Liver
Kidney
Spleen
Kidney
Spine

Intestines
Intestines
Transverse colon

Descending colon

Sigmoid colon

Ascending colon
Transverse colon

The foot maps: 3-5 year olds
By the age of about 3 the feet begin to change shape, with a distinctive narrowing caused by the formation of the arches. This is an important clue for the reflexologist, who can now identify the middle of the body at the narrowing point of each foot: this is the reflex line of the transverse colon.

The feet are still too small for the kind of precise treatment that is possible in later years. Nonetheless, these simplified maps provide a broad but useful indication of the principal divisions. As the foot develops the main guidelines – at the diaphragm, waist, and pelvis – become clearer (see pp. 12-13).

Comforting your baby

Regular treatments of the whole foot make an important contribution to the baby's general wellbeing. However, certain common ailments of babyhood respond well to more concentrated work on one or more of the areas in the working drawings below, which also show how to work the whole foot, as described on p. 52.

After a traumatic birth...

If your baby was born by forceps delivery, or if the labour was very long, you can help offset the trauma of this uncomfortable way of entering the world by working, from the word go, on your baby's feet.

Cranial osteopathy is also considered beneficial in these circumstances. Arrange, if you can, for the osteopath to visit you, in home or in hospital, soon after the birth.

Reflexology treatment
As well as giving frequent general treaments, concentrate on the spine as well as the head and neck areas (see p. 55). This will help improve the circulation to those areas under particular stress at the time of the birth. Do this for a minute or so every time you pick up your baby.

Calming colic

The main cause of excessive crying in the first few weeks of life is colic, said to be caused by an immature digestive system. Babies who are born prematurely with a low

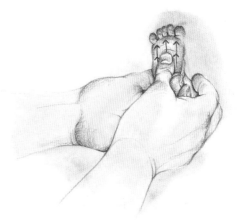

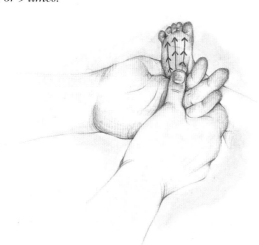

Working the digestive system: 1
Supporting the right foot with your left hand, use your right thumb to work over the entire heel area. Do this gently, 2 or 3 times.

Working the digestive system: 2
Still maintaining only gentle pressure, move up to work across the middle area of the foot, from the inside to the outside edge. Repeat both steps on the left foot.

birth weight, and those whose passage into the world was traumatic, seem prone to it.

Reflexology treatment
Evening colic is common in the first 8 weeks or so and treating the foot for 5 minutes or so may help to relieve it. Work from the base of the heel to where the toes join the foot, covering the digestive and intestinal areas (see p. 54). Improving circulation to these parts helps both absorption and elimination.

Do not be surprised if you hear a lot of rumbling and gurgling in the abdominal area. This is a sign of increased muscular activity in the stomach and bowel, which should reduce the pain of colic, caused by "trapped wind" in the lower bowel.

Support Strategies
Colic
Breastfeeding mothers *can help calm colic while stimulating their milk supply by drinking strong infusions of camomile, cinnamon, cardamom, or fennel. Traces of these herbs or spices, which are also good for digestion, will be passed on via the breast milk, helping the baby's digestion in a natural way.*

Camomile tea *may be given to babies over 3 months who are still suffering from colic. It is soothing for the digestion and is obtainable from most pharmacies in a form especially prepared for babies.*

Working the head and neck areas
Supporting the top of the tiny foot with your left thumb, apply gentle pressure to the general area beneath and over the toes. Repeat on the left foot.

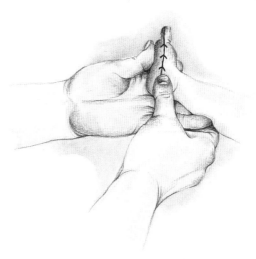

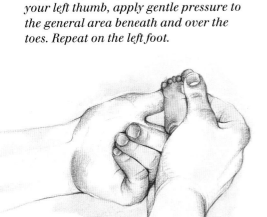

Working the spine
Support the right foot with your left hand, as shown, and work the spine reflexes along the side of the foot up to the top of the big toe. Repeat on the left foot.

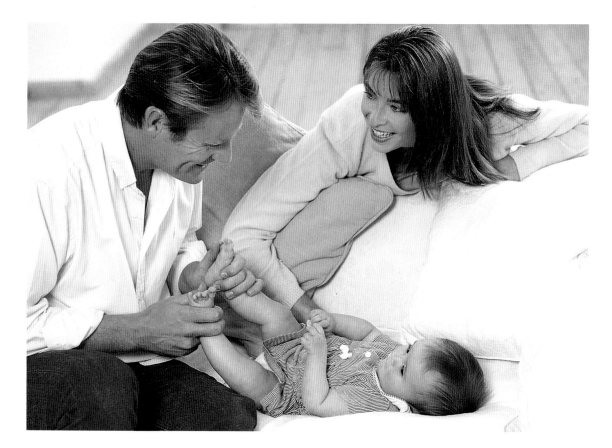

Cradle cap and allergies

Babies with cradle cap are more likely to develop some form of allergic reactive condition in their early years. Be on the lookout for typical signs, such as sneezing, hyperactivity, skin irritations, and the tendency to produce excessive mucus, which may lead to frequent upper and lower respiratory tract infections.

Warm olive oil, left on overnight and washed off the following day, helps loosen the scales that form primarily on the scalp.

Reflexology treatment
Working the digestive system on a regular basis helps strengthen it. This should help reduce the likelihood of the baby developing an allergic condition (see also pp. 116-117).

Stimulating sleepy feeders

Some new-born babies find it hard to feed for more than a few minutes without falling asleep. They then wake again an hour or so later for another short feed. The young first-time mother may thus find herself constantly feeding. If the baby is being breast fed, frequent suckling makes the nipples painful and the breasts may become engorged.

Reflexology treatment
Work up the foot from the heel to the base of the toes as described on p. 52, but this time using tiny circling movements. This stimulation should make the baby more alert and capable of taking in sufficient quantities of milk to allow for an interval of 3 or 4 hours before the next feed.

The joy of having created a child is one of life's "peak experiences." Loving, playful, physical contact in the early months has a unique quality that cannot be recaptured in later life.

Teething troubles

The eruption of teeth causes many babies much distress and discomfort, often with feverish symptoms. It is important that signs of more serious conditions are not mistaken for teething. A child who is feverish, with heightened colour in the face, generally below par, and refusing food is probably fighting off some infection. If symptoms persist for more than 24 hours it would be wise to get professional advice.

Reflexology treatment
The goal of treatment is to calm the child and reduce the temperature. Gentle work on the whole foot should soothe babies; for infants, the relaxing exercises described on pp.24-25 can be given before treating the foot.

Support Strategies
Teething troubles
Give the baby something to chew on that does not break easily

*A **high liquid** intake is essential for babies and children – or indeed anyone – with a fever. Offer bottled water or natural (diluted) fruit juices as well as milk.*

Camomile tea with honey is soothing in feverish states. Not only is honey a healing food, it may help bowel action if the fever has caused constipation.

John: 3 months, with sleeping & feeding problems

John was just 12 weeks old when his parents decided to try reflexology as an alternative approach in their efforts to help their baby become more content. He had been fretful from birth, perhaps because of his traumatic entry into the world by forceps delivery. He slept little, fed badly, and seemed to have problems with colic, particularly in the evenings. In addition, he was frequently constipated and was underweight. Needless to say, his young parents found all this deeply worrying and wearing. The local clinic had offered advice and help, but nothing worked.

I started giving John regular treatments, just working out the whole of the sole of each foot. Five minutes on each was plenty. And since daily treatments are of such benefit, I taught the parents how to work his feet. I also advised them to give him an ounce or so of camomile tea each day, since it is soothing for the digestive system.

His parents reported at the second appointment that shortly after working on John's feet, loud rumbling sounds came from his stomach, followed by a normal bowel action.

At the next appointment I again gave John a reflexology treatment, this time following it with a light massage with baby oil on his lower back and abdominal area.

We continued working as a team, with daily treatments reinforced by a weekly visit to my clinic. After just 6 sessions, the crying ceased, John began to smile, his constipation was much improved, and for the first time in his life he began to sleep for 6 hours at night. To the amazement of his parents (and the local health clinic), he began to gain weight, looked much healthier, and, rather than being restless and fretful, was clearly contented.

Treating children's ailments

Reflexology is effective in alleviating the symptoms of certain common ailments in early childhood. Many of these occur equally in adults, but this chapter suggests ways of treating them that are appropriate for young children. If you do not find what you are looking for here, consult pp. 72-119.

Asthma
In the polluted air of modern cities, children are suffering more and more from asthma. Reflexology may help reduce the severity or frequency of attacks. See pp. 88-89.

Chest infections
Because the respiratory tract in the very young is much narrower than in an adult, it becomes congested more readily. Babies, who have not learned to cough or blow their nose to help clear the air passages, make particularly heavy weather out of colds.

Reflexology treatment
This should bring some relief by helping drain the sinuses as well as improving immunity. Work first on the right foot and then on the left, concentrating on the upper part of the foot where the lung and chest reflexes are found.

See p. 90 for treating more mature feet.

Support Strategies

Stop smoking! *Children's health suffers from passive smoking. NB Not smoking in front of them does **not** count as not exposing children to smoke.*

Humidify *the air by hanging water containers on central heating radiators.*

Sprinkle decongestant oils *on pillows or use them in vaporizers overnight.*

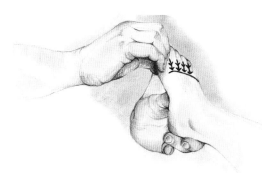

2 Work the lung and chest (top)
Support the right foot with your left hand, as shown, and use your right index finger to work down the grooves on top of the foot. Repeat on the left foot.

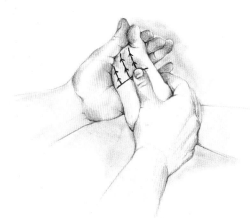

1 Work the lung and chest (sole)
Supporting the right foot with your left hand, use your right thumb to work up each area from the diaphragm line to the base of each toe. Repeat on the left foot.

Constipation

This problem in adult life may have had its roots in childhood. Constipation in children is usually due to a combination of poor diet and lack of exercise: the intestinal area is a convoluted tube activated by strong muscle movements, which are stimulated by food and encouraged by physical activity.

Being ferried to and from school by car, often forbidden to roam the fields or play outdoors unsupervised, and only too inclined to spend long hours immobile in front of a tv set, some young children miss out on the physical activity that encourages regular bowel function.

A good breakfast should stimulate a bowel action. Make sure your child gets up early enough to eat in an unhurried way and to have time for a bowel movement before leaving the house. Many children are reluctant to use communal school facilities for this, and suppress the need all day until they come home. This "holding on" is to be discouraged, not least because it establishes bad habits which may continue into later life.

Reflexology treatment
Stimulate the intestinal area, repeating the procedure described below several times on each foot. The child will probably have a bowel action shortly after treatment.

If the foot has begun to narrow, you can treat the intestinal area more precisely, and instructions on treating more mature feet are given on p. 103. In the under 3 year olds, simply concentrate generally on the intestinal area. Treatment should be offered, if possible, on a daily basis.

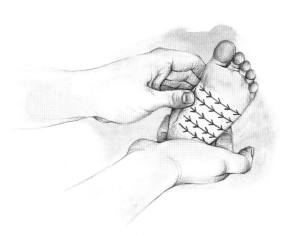

Working the intestinal area
Work the area shown on both feet. The drawing shows work on the left foot, using the left thumb to work the whole area from the middle of the foot to the base of the heel.

Support Strategies

Explain to your children *that cleaning the inside of the body is as important as cleaning the outside. Encourage them to drink plenty of water every day.*

Diet *Make sure their diet includes plenty of roughage in the form of wholegrain (not bran-based) breakfast cereals, dried fruits, raisins, wholemeal bread, and raw vegetables. Cut up into fingers, the latter are fun to eat.*

Regularity *of bowel movements can be encouraged by getting children to use the toilet at a regular time each day. The bowel performs well to a daily routine. But don't allow regularity to become an obsession.*

Croup

Children have a narrower trachea (airway) than adults, and when this area becomes inflamed, it narrows still further, possibly becoming so small that there is a danger of suffocation.

A harsh barking cough and difficulty in breathing, often at night, are symptoms of this distressing condition, the causes of which include viral or bacterial infections, particularly in the winter months.

Putting the child in a steamy atmosphere – by running hot water in the shower or bathtub to fill the room with steam, or by boiling kettles full of water – is the traditional first aid measure, aimed at relieving congestion and making breathing easier.

If this treatment does not help, and the child is struggling to breathe and starting to go bluish around the lips, you must seek immediate medical attention at the nearest hospital emergency department.

Difficult as it may be to remain calm in the face of such frightening symptoms, it is

Earache

The eustachian tube, which joins the throat to the ear, is very narrow in young children. For this reason ear infections are common in babies and in the under fives, often accompanying a simple cold. The pain is extreme and parents should always seek medical advice. Most ear infections are not bacterial in origin, so there is no urgent need for antibiotics. However, if the pain continues for more than 48 hours, the doctor may prescribe them.

Reflexology treatment
This may provide some relief from pain. The ear reflexes are on the third toe of each foot, but since it is difficult to find the exact spot on a very small foot, just apply pressure to the whole area of the third toe.

Working the heart reflex
This reflex only occurs on the left foot. Support the foot with your right hand and use your left thumb to work the area shown. In children, as in adults, it is important not to overwork this area.

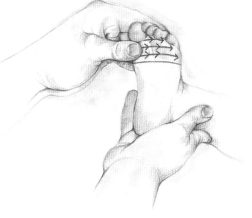

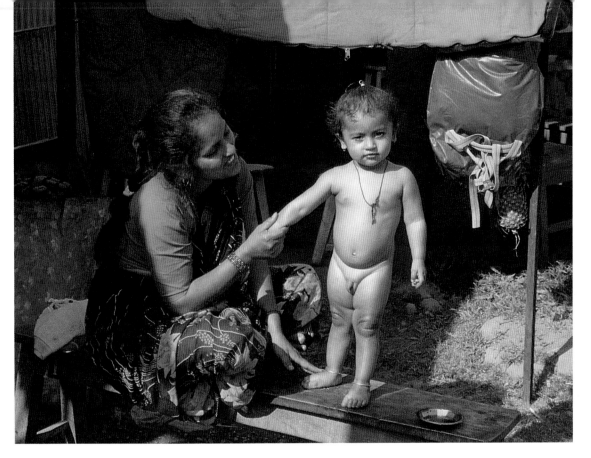

*A **Nepalese mother**, interrupted in her morning massage of her baby son, instinctively maintains contact with him, holding foot and hand so that the energy circle remains unbroken. A tiny metal dish holds the massage oil.*

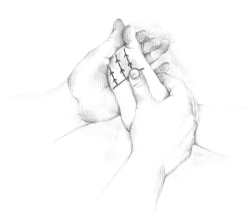

Working the lung reflex (sole)
Supporting the right foot with your left hand, use your right thumb to work over the area shown. Then work over the top of the foot as shown on p. 58.

essential that you do so, for your child's sake. Comfort and reassurance are what the child needs at times like this. Any signs of panic on your part can only serve to exacerbate the situation. Whatever you do to help, including getting the child to the hospital, do it with as much quiet assurance as you can muster.

Reflexology treatment
Croup occurs most frequently in children under the age of 4. Treatment is preventive in that it aims to strengthen the child's respiratory system. Treat the heart and lung areas at the top of the feet, weekly.

Eczema

This distressing skin disorder causes dry, scaly, or weeping skin that may be red, painful, and extremely irritating. Eczema runs in families and is common in those where there is a history of asthma, hay fever, and general skin sensitivity.

Stress usually aggravates symptoms, so it is not unusual for the skin to flare up when the child is faced with situations outside the normal daily routine. Milestones such as the introduction to nursery school or the start of full-time schooling, for example, may provoke outbreaks of eczema.

Reflexology treatment
Gentle treatments, starting with the relaxation exercises (see pp. 24-25) to induce a state of calmness, can be given well in advance to prepare the child to cope with a potentially stressful situation.

Work on the digestive system is important and beneficial in helping the body cope with an allergic state. For working a baby's feet, see p. 54. Treating the digestive areas in young children is explained on p. 59. For older children, follow the instructions for allergies on pp. 116-117.

Temper tantrums

These expressions of extreme frustration usually begin around the age of 2 and last until about the age of 4, when the child becomes more articulate. Much as parents may appreciate that uncontrolled outbursts of screaming and rage may arise from the child's inability to explain a need or wish, such outbursts are, to say the least, very difficult to cope with.

On an immediate practical level, it pays to be prepared, and to take steps to mitigate or avoid those situations that usually provoke a tantrum. There may, however, be more to temper tantrums than ungratified wishes. Children who suffer from them are often also more susceptible to hyperactivity (see p. 66). And since food additives are strongly implicated in hyperactivity, it makes sense to wean a child prone to tantrums off those foods that contain quantities of colourings and chemicals.

Cola drinks, artificial fruit juices, highly coloured confectionery, and ice lollipops (particularly those with yellow and orange colouring), and chocolate have all been associated with extreme and inappropriate behaviour in young children.

Reflexology treatment
The principal goal, if an allergy is suspected, is to help the elimination of toxins by working on the liver, the kidneys, bowel, and bladder. On a small foot, treat the entire digestive area, as shown on p. 59. In addition to this, help the child to become more relaxed generally by starting each session with the foot-relaxing routine (pp. 24-25).

Skin care

Don't use soap; instead use a soap-free cleanser.

◆

Add a little oil, such as soya oil, to the child's bath, and use oatmeal to gently scrub the skin. Baths are soothing, though they may be aggravating at first. NB If you use oil in the bath, make sure the child doesn't slip.

◆

Use a good lanolin moisturizer, if it suits you, to keep the skin well moisturized – an important measure.

Support Strategies

Eczema

Furry or woollen toys, though much loved, may be best set aside. A lot of eczema sufferers are sensitive to wool.

Avoid biological washing powders and fabric softeners. Double rinse clothes.

Use hypo-allergenic pillows and mattress covers.

House mite allergy If you notice that the eczema flares up after the child has been crawling on the floor, mites could be the cause of the problem.

Problem foods that may provoke allergic reactions include dairy products, wheat, sugars, orange, red, and purple fruits, as well as food colourings and additives. Try to identify the culprits by keeping an allergy diary, as shown on p. 116.

Tonsillitis

This common complaint occurs most frequently in children under 9. Sore throat, aches and pains, loss of appetite, and fever are frequent symptoms. If they continue for more than 48 hours, seek medical advice.

Reflexology treatment
Work over the head and neck areas at the top of the foot and over the toes, to reduce pain. Also work the intestines (see p. 59) to contact the spleen, and help to strengthen the immune system. For instructions on working more mature feet see p. 84.

Melanie: 7 years old with weakness in limbs

Minor brain damage at birth meant that Melanie had a severe weakness in her right leg and arm. She dragged her leg, which meant that she had many falls, and this prevented her joining in physical games and activities with her schoolfriends. She had been receiving physiotherapy, but now, at the age of 7, it was decided that little more could be achieved.

Melanie's parents had heard about reflexology, and came to me to see if treatment might improve their daughter's mobility. I began weekly treatments, and showed her parents how to treat the crucial spinal area to stimulate the central nervous system and the brain on a daily basis.

Melanie showed no signs of improvement at all in the first 2 months, although she really enjoyed the treatment. However, at the end of the third month, her parents noticed that a week had passed without her falling, and they hardly dared mention the fact that she seemed to have more control over her leg.

We all continued with reflexology and at the end of 9 months of constant treatment Melanie's walking was so improved that her original problem was hardly noticeable. The consultant at the local hospital was astonished at the unexpected improvement. When her parents excitedly explained the role of reflexology, he confessed: "I'm afraid I really don't know anything about reflexology, but my advice to you is to just keep on with this treatment. The improvement is amazing."

Stressful reactions in children

The adult assertion that "Schooldays are the happiest days of your life" is likely to be greeted with groans of disbelief and protest from those who know better. Parents, clinging to a rosy vision of times past, often fail to recall or recognize the stresses, strains, and upheavals of childhood. And, even if they do recognize them, they often feel powerless to help, or assume that problems will be dealt with, somehow, by teachers or other professionals.

Childhood has more than its share of traumatic events, any of which may provoke a stressful reaction in the child – from bedwetting to nightmares. Ongoing unhappiness may lead to overeating, or a tendency to be accident prone.

Since siblings are more likely to be able to relate to one another's problems, part of this chapter (pp. 70-71)) is addressed to young people. If your children are likely to be interested, suggest that they take time to read this short explanation of how reflexology can be used to help relieve some of the difficult situations in which they or their friends may find themselves. Regular reflexology sessions bring parents and children closer together, allowing precious opportunities for discussion and airing of problems. As a parent, do not force the issue, but gently encourage your child to talk about their preoccupations, fears, and anxieties.

Children as reflexologists
The beauty of reflexology – apart from its effectivenes – is its simplicity. Young children, who tend to be very much in touch with their feelings and those of other people, are quick to learn and can be encouraged from an early age to give one or two simple treatments.

They can work not only on their siblings, but on adults. The child who is able to give a visiting grandparent a tonic treatment to help alleviate the pain of an arthritic shoulder, for example, is empowered by that experience. Usually on the receiving end as far as adults are concerned, the child has an opportunity to give loving help to an older person, and to see the positive results of that giving.

Stress and disease
Stress depletes the body's immune system and resistance to disease. It is also responsible for triggering many debilitating conditions, particularly those related to the digestive and respiratory systems. Certain other conditions of childhood, though not specifically recognized as illnesses, may signal a "dis-ease" in the child. Treatment for some of the more common ones is discussed in this section. With reflexology, as with other holistic treatments, the aim is to treat the cause and not the symptoms.

Accident-prone children
The child who always seems to have a leg in plaster, an arm in a sling, or a bandage around the head is often dismissed, with a sigh, as being "accident prone."

One school of thought, however, suggests that such accidents are not due to mere clumsiness but to an unconscious strategy to win attention. So, if one of your offspring is accident prone, and you have checked that there is no obvious physical cause, it is worth taking a close look at your family lifestyle to see if the child in question is getting enough of your time – and by this is meant "quality" time and attention.

In large families, for example, where children as young as 7 or 8 may take a

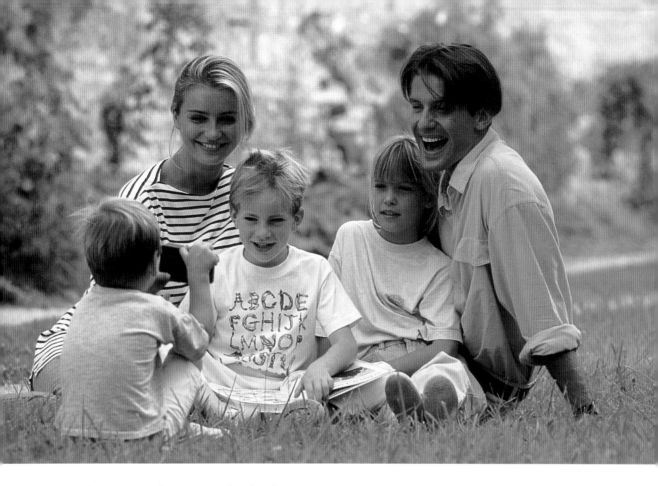

considerable amount of responsibilty for the care of younger siblings, it is important to ensure that their own needs for nurturing are met – that they are not always greeted by a baby at the breast when they themselves want a cuddle on mother's lap.

If both parents are working and return tired at the end of the day it needs a special effort to set aside a time, in addition to doing the cooking and attending to household chores, to simply sit and be with the children, to listen to them.

The physical communication and warmth of contact of reflexology could be the solution to a lot of hurts. Somehow just taking their feet into your hands seems to unlock the mind of the receiver, and in the relaxed state that reflexology induces a child may readily share fears and anxieties. If there are several children in the family,

Having fun together as a family is a joy beyond price and essential for the rounded, happy development of each child. Try not to let pressures of work reduce these times of interaction.

parents can share the treating – in such a way that each parent spends a little time with each child once or twice a week.

Remember that communication such as this does not call for words. If neither you nor your child wishes to talk, simply enjoy a loving silence.

Reflexology treatment
For general wellbeing, work on both feet from the base of the heel up to the area where the toes join the feet, with small forward creeping movements. Also work out the area of the spine, found on the inside edge of both feet (see pp. 14-15).

Bedwetting

Before the age of 5 bedwetting is not considered a problem. After that age, lack of bladder control at night may be due to a deep-seated anxiety or to the fact that the child is sleeping so deeply that he or she is unaware of the natural signals from the bladder to empty its contents. Take professional advice to make sure that there is no medical reason, such as a urinary infection, for the problem, before using reflexology to supplement other common sense measures. These include lifting the child at intervals through the night and cutting out fluids for a couple of hours before bedtime.

Reflexology treatment
Give the child a treatment every night before bed. First use all the relaxation exercises (see pp. 24-25), then, to help the bladder function generally, work out the bladder and ureter on both feet.

If the foot is small, work the area indicated on p. 59. On older children, treat the same area as for adults, see p. 16.

Support Strategies
for bedwetting
Cinnamon bark is a traditional remedy. Get your child to chew on a piece at intervals during the day, or sprinkle some powder in hot milk and sweeten it.

Diet Cut out cola and chocolate drinks, as well as drinks and sweets (candies) containing yellow or orange food colouring. All have been associated with bedwetting.

Support Strategies
for hyperactivity
Camomile tea has a sedative effect and is safe to give to children of any age.

Supplements that may help are: vitamin B complex (or a multivitamin formulated for children) and evening primrose oil (50 mg per 6 kg/1 stone in weight). Do not give the latter if the child has fits.

Food cravings in a hyperactive child should be viewed with extreme suspicion. If, for example, the child is always taking cheese from the refrigerator or sugar from the bowl, make these foodstuffs top of your list of allergy suspects. Then take steps to identify them, and eliminate them by keeping an allergy diary (see p. 116).

Hyperactive children

An important first step when trying to get to the root of hyperactivity in young children is to look at their diet, since hyperactivity may be associated with an allergic reaction. Certain drinks, particularly those containing artificial sweeteners, colouring agents, and caffeine, are known to have a stimulating effect. Dairy products, orange, red, and purple fruits, wheat, yeasts, and sugars also commonly cause allergic reactions.

Reflexology treatment
To calm the child in periods of excitability, concentrate on the highly beneficial relaxation exercises (see pp. 24-25).

Treat on a regular basis those areas of the foot related to the intestines, since allergic reactions are often related to a weaknes in the digestive system. You can treat the area generally in the under 5 year old (see p. 59). For older children, follow the digestive system treatment outlined on pp. 100-101. For more detailed discussion of allergies, see pp. 116-117.

Nightmares

Frightening real-life experiences as well as deep-seated anxieties and fears may be expressed in nightmares or night terrors. The only immediate treatment is to comfort the child, reassuring him or her that it is only a dream. If night terrors persist, seek professional guidance.

Reflexology treatment
Soothe the child before bedtime with the foot relaxation exercises (see pp. 24-25). The diaphragm relaxation is particularly beneficial since it puts the body into the correct mode for sleep.

see pp. 100-101 / see pp. 116-117 / see p. 59 / see pp. 24-25

Support Strategies
for nightmares
The last meal of the day should be taken at least 3 hours before bedtime, to allow time for digestion before going to bed.

Control TV viewing generally and check particularly on the suitability of pre-bedtime shows.

A warm milk drink with half a teaspoon of nutmeg and 1 or 2 teaspoons of honey helps induce sleep.

Support Strategies
for obesity
Diet Seek medical advice, if necessary, on a balanced, healthy, non-fattening diet (see p. 41).

A gentle exercise programme, that the child is interested in, should complement dietary changes.

Encourage sensible snacks, such as celery or carrot sticks. Discourage crisps (chips), chocolate, etc.

Forbid fad diets!

Counselling may help both parents and children in defining and dealing with the basic cause of over-eating.

Obesity in children

The most common causes of obesity in children – until recently an essentially western complaint – are the over-consumption of high-calorie foods and lack of exercise. Only rarely is there a "glandular" disturbance at the root of the problem.

Parents are responsible for their children's eating habits, which are laid down in infancy. It may be, of course, that the problem reflects the family's normal eating habits, with too great an emphasis on carbohydrates, and it can be corrected with a change to a more healthy diet (see p. 41).

On the other hand, an overindulgence in confectionery or high-calorie fast foods, which are aggressively advertised on television, could be symptomatic of an inner tension or unhappiness.

In a large family, for example, if one child is overweight, it is likely to be the one who is neglected, perhaps bearing responsibility for siblings but missing out on parental attention.

Eating may also compensate for feelings of inadequacy, insecurity, or inferiority; indulgence in high-calorie foods, especially chocolate, gives a temporary "lift" and this indulgence soon becomes a habit. Since being overweight means that exercising is not easy, a vicious circle is set up in which the child puts on increasing amounts of weight and resorts more and more to food as a source of solace.

Reflexology treatment
This can help not only by relaxing and soothing tensions, but by allowing the parents to focus loving attention on the individual child, and to listen attentively to any worries he or she wants to share.

Children love the relaxation treatments, so begin a session by offering these (see pp. 24-25) before going on to work the central nervous system, concentrating on the spine and brain areas as shown below.

Travel (motion) sickness

Long journeys by road, sea, or air are not easy with young children, and if one of the younger members of the party is prone to travel sickness, such journeys can be exceptionally gruelling (all round!). Children are likely to suffer particularly from car sickness, which is sometimes associated with particular kinds of road surfaces. Fortunately they usually grow out of it as they get older.

Reflexology treatment
Since the symptoms of travel sickness – nausea, vomiting, or faintness – are linked to an oversensitivity of the inner ear, work the ear reflex before setting out on a long journey. To do this, support the right foot with your left hand and use your right thumb to make small circular, clockwise movements on the crease at the top of the third toe where it bends. Work over this

1 Work the spine
Support the top of the right foot with your left hand. Use your right thumb to work along the spinal reflexes on the inside edge. Repeat on the left foot.

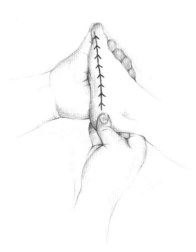

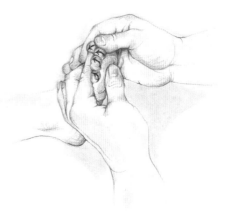

2 Work the brain
Supporting the right foot with your left hand, use your right thumb to work over the very top of the first three toes. Repeat on the left foot.

reflex several times before changing hands and working on the left foot.

If the child's foot is too small for you to locate this small point, work the hand instead, treating the entire length of the middle finger on both hands. The child could treat this same area him- or herself while travelling – an effective form of self-help as well as a welcome diversionary tactic. Preventive treatment may also help dispel anxiety based on previous attacks, in itself a frequent trigger of travel sickness.

Support Strategies

Before the journey

A light meal is all the child needs. A full stomach, or even just the sight of food, can make things worse.

Ginger tea taken in small but regular doses before and during the journey helps settle the stomach. Make your own from a piece of ginger root, or buy it ready made. Take a flask with you on the journey.
Passiflora is a herbal remedy that has a calming effect. One tablet should be taken 2 hours before setting out.

◆

During the journey

Sucking boiled sweets(hard candy) helps, and this medicinal use of sugar is allowable!
Stuffy, smoky atmospheres make things worse. Avoid them. In a car, open the windows.
Devise games (number plate spotting, cow counting, or word games) as distractions.

The turbulent teens

The teenage years can be traumatic for parents as well as for their offspring. As the young person struggles to come to terms with profound emotional and physical changes, including strongly emerging sexuality, parents who hitherto have felt confident about their ability to help and comfort their offspring often find themselves at a loss. Only too keenly conscious of their child's mood swings, withdrawal, or painful obsession with personal appearance, their attempts at sympathy or understanding often meet with rejection.

The teenager is not only going through a virtual metamorphosis physically, but is also, probably, in the throes of an identity crisis. Keen for independence, their rejection of their parents and their values may be fierce.

The role of reflexology
As in so many other situations of emotional upheaval, a reflexology treatment "speaks louder than words." A teenager who is feeling angry and alienated from the rest of the family recognizes, through the healing hands-on treatment offered by a parent or sibling, that that person cares and sympathizes. In the United States, professional reflexologists enlisted to work with teenagers receiving help for alcohol or drug abuse report impressive results.

The major contribution of reflexology is to reduce the high levels of stress experienced in the teens. If by reducing stress, it also leads to a reduction in outbreaks of acne, it will be a particularly welcome treatment. Make the general foot relaxation exercises (pp. 24-25) a regular routine and work the endocrine system (see pp. 108-109) in an attempt to redress the balance at a time of considerable hormonal upheaval.

A postscript for older children...

As you get older, and begin to explore beyond the close family circle, life seems to contain more and more "significant" events. Your first day at nursery school was one of these, and you may remember it as an exciting or an anxious time, or a mixture of both. You probably experienced similar mixed feelings when you moved on to junior and then senior school, when you joined the scouts, or were chosen for the tennis team.

Going out into the world
Feeling anxious at first about new, unknown situations is normal. Once you have had a while to get used to them, you begin to feel relaxed and secure. Nonetheless, as your circle of friends and acquaintances gets wider, you almost inevitably encounter problems with relationships, in much the same way as adults do. Your best friend may go off with another, leaving you feeling rejected and miserable. You may be fearful of walking home alone from school in case you are set upon by a gang of bullies. School itself may bring its own set of problems, as you worry about your course work or approaching examinations.

On the emotional roller coaster
There are all kinds of emotional ups and downs associated with the simple fact of maturing, physically and mentally. You may become obsessed with and self-conscious about an aspect of your physical appearance that you dislike. You may feel deep irritation or anger toward your parents. Or you may just feel generally low – for no apparent reason, you have got the "blues." These uncomfortable feelings are an unavoidable part of growing up for most people.

A feeling of isolation may make matters worse. You don't want to talk to your parents but feel your brothers or sisters would not understand either.

The power of silence
There are times, though, when words are unnecessary. When feelings can be expressed and understood in other ways. One way is through touch. If you come from a family where people hug each other a lot, where touching is a normal part of your lives, then you already know how comforting it is.

If physical contact is rare, you may feel embarrassed or uncomfortable about displaying emotion in this way.

Give reflexology a go!
Reflexology provides you with a safe, acceptable way of making caring contact with other people. So, if you don't feel much like talking to your parents, at least allow them to work on your feet. Or offer to give someone a relaxing foot massage yourself.

Treat your brothers and sisters
Suppose, for example, that your younger sister has come home from school in tears because she hasn't been invited to a friend's party. Why not offer her a reflexolgy session, to help her calm down, and maybe give her a chance to talk about how she feels?

When you're moody...
Mood swings in puberty are caused by the hormonal changes taking place in your body. If you are a girl, one day you may be longing to be grown up, wearing a bra, makeup, and trendy clothes; the next you are back playing with your dolls. If you are feeling inexplicably irritated or low, get a brother or

sister to give you a relaxing reflexology treatment!

...or heartbroken

Puberty is the time when relationships with members of the opposite sex become very important. If you are heartbroken because the love of your life has dropped you, get someone in your family to give you a treatment. A brother or sister with whom you can share your feelings is probably the best person. Similarly, don't hesitate to offer treatment if you see that they are miserable.

Facing nerve-wracking events

The very thought of impending examinations can create all manner of anxieties. As the dreaded day approaches, you may find yourself suffering from an increased need to urinate, attacks of diarrhea, or even panic attacks. All this is due to the increase of adrenaline in your bloodstream. This is the "fight or flight" hormone that is released in greater quantities in times of crisis.

A reflexology treatment the night before the examination, interview, or other major event will encourage calm and a good night's sleep, enabling you to perform as best you can the next day.

Don't forget the "wrinklies!"

You need not restrict your reflexology treatments to the younger members of your family. Be on the alert for times when one of your parents could do with some attention, perhaps when they are worried or overworked. And if an arthritic grandparent comes to visit, offer them a treatment.

Always remember that reflexology is as satisfying for the giver as for the receiver.

Amy: 15 years old with tinnitus

Amy was brought to my surgery by her parents. She suffered from constant ringing in her ears, or tinnitus. Specialist examination of her ears had revealed no abnormality.

I was immediately aware of the tension in her parents, who had had Amy, an only child, in their late 40s. Our first appointment was far from relaxed. Her parents answered all the questions directed at Amy, and I could see the pain this caused her.

At the second appointment I asked her parents to remain in the waiting room. As I treated her, Amy unwound, revealing that her parents spent most of the time arguing and that this had been going on for as long as she could remember. Her mother suffered from migraines, and her father had high blood pressure.

After 3 reflexology sessions, there was no improvement in Amy's ears, though by now I suspected that her tinnitus was an unconscious attempt to block out an intolerable family situation. I nervously broached this with her parents, who were upset but went away to ponder the suggestion.

With the help of a book and some instruction from me, Amy began to treat her own hands between sessions. I suggested that she also practise on her parents. The treatments worked remarkably in breaking down family tensions. Gradually, not only did Amy's tinnitus subside, but so did her parents' arguing. Her parents then decided to come for treatment as well: in 8 weeks her mother's migraines had ceased and her father's blood pressure had dropped. Within 3 months, Amy's tinnitus had disappeared.

Chapter Four

Treating Adult Ailments

From top to toe – from migraines to chilblains – reflexology can help alleviate the symptoms as well as prevent the recurrence of many common ailments.

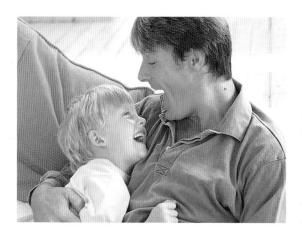

Reflexology sessions can be fun *for all the family. Try to make sure everyone gets a complete foot workout once a week, on a "maintenance" basis, to ensure their continuing good health. Prevention is always better than cure, so, though it does offer quick relief in some situations, resist the temptation to reach for reflexology as you might for a bottle of aspirin.*

Reflexology has a good track record in treating all of the common ailments included in this chapter. They are grouped according to the part of the body in which they occur – working from top to toe. Since time is often at a premium, the treatments concentrate solely on those reflexes immediately involved in each condition. Step-by-step drawings, with working areas clearly indicated, are accompanied by easy-to-follow instructions. Intersperse all treatments with those foot relaxation exercises (pp. 24-25) that particularly appeal to the receiver.

Restoring balance in the digestive (pp. 100-101) and endocrine (pp. 108-109) systems is a prime requirement in so many conditions (many of them stress-related) that these "key" systems are set out in their entirety. There is separate discussion, too, of allergies (pp. 116-117) and arthritis (pp. 118-119), both of which may be manifest in several different parts of the body.

Readers who wish to work on their own hands are referred to the relevant pages of the complete hand workout (pp. 32-37).

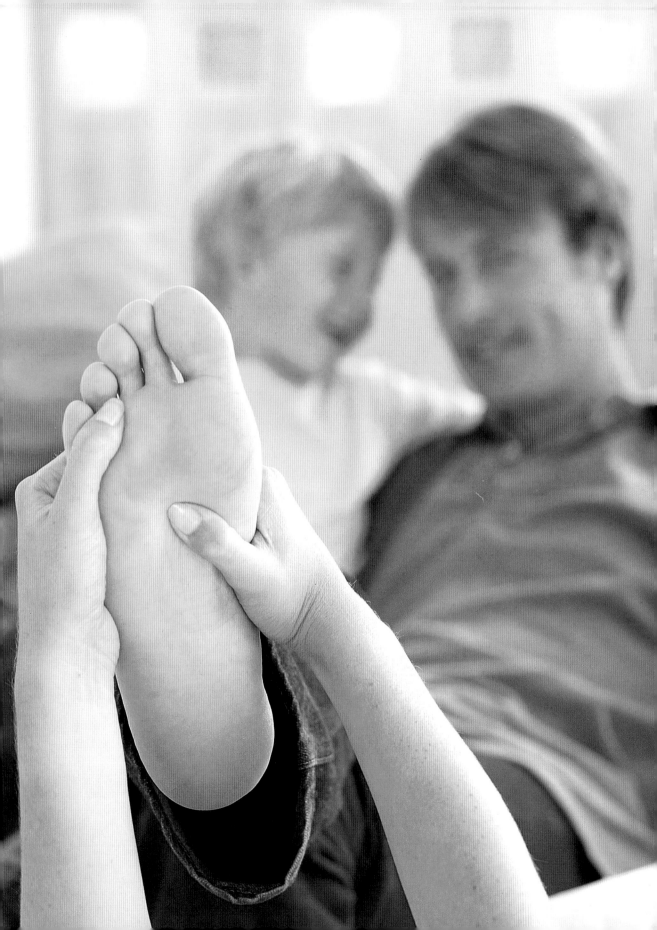

Treating the head & neck areas

Headaches and migraine

There may be an obvious physical reason for a headache – too many hours in front of a computer monitor, a stuffy atmosphere, or a hangover, for example. Other common causes of headaches are worry and anxiety, which give rise to physical tension, often in the neck. Migraine, though often related to overwork or stress, may also be directly linked to a food allergy.

Reflexology treatment
For headaches with a known physical cause, treat the spine, concentrating on the neck area at the top of the spine, to release tension. For stress-related headaches and neck problems (including cricks, stiffness, and whiplash injury), treat the brain as well as the cervical spine, giving 1 or 2 treatments daily, interspersed with the general foot relaxation exercises (see pp. 24-25).

Since migraine often seems to be related to the digestion, improving liver function and reducing stress are the main goals. Treat the sufferer frequently in the passive periods: 2 or 3 times a week for about 3 months should produce positive results. Work the brain and cervical spine areas, and then concentrate on the liver reflex.

**Self-help:
working your own hands
*for headaches, work***
1 The brain (*see p. 34*)
2 The cervical spine (*see p. 34*)
for migraine, work 1, 2, plus
3 The liver (*see p. 35*)

1 Work the brain
Support the right foot with your left hand. Use your right thumb to work over the tops of the first 3 toes, starting with the big toe. If the headache is acute and this area is extra sensitive, use only a light pressure.

Treat for about 5 minutes. Repeat on the left foot.

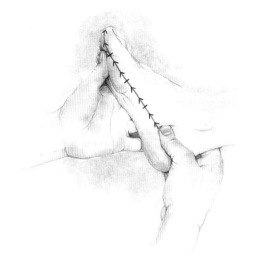

2 Work the cervical spine

Support the right foot with your left hand. With your right thumb, work up the spine reflex. Then concentrate on the cervical spine area on the inside edge of the big toe, starting at the point where the toe joins the foot. Repeat on the left foot.

After working the spine, use the ankle-freeing exercise (see p. 24).

After working the spine, use the ankle-freeing exercise (see p. 24).

3 Work the liver

For migraine, work this in addition to steps 1 and 2. Support the top of the right foot with your left hand and use your right thumb to treat the area indicated from the inside to the outside edge of the foot. Then work back in the opposite direction. (Right foot only.)

Support Strategies

Headaches

Drink *plenty of water.*

Make a cold compress, *lie down with it across your eyes and gently go through one of the relaxation techniques described on pp. 42-43.*

Massage *may help to release tension and ease pain in the head and neck. Use pure almond oil or blend it with a few drops of lavender oil. Make soothing light strokes around the neck, shoulders, and over the upper spine.*

Migraine

Identify triggers *by keeping a migraine diary. See Allergies, pp. 116-117.*

Feverfew *is a helpful prophylactic. Take 50-60mg daily, 14 days on and 14 days off.*

Cayenne in lemon juice *sounds gruesome, but is worth taking in the morning to ward off migraine if you anticipate a stressful day. Mix a quarter teaspoon of cayenne powder with the juice of half a lemon. Add to a tumbler of warm water and drink it quickly!*

Avoid *stress-inducing situations.*

Treating ear problems
Earache, tinnitus

Alleviating earache
It is important to seek medical advice promptly about all pains in the ear. They may be due to an infection either of the middle or outer ear. Middle-ear infections are usually accompanied by cold-type symptoms. Those of the outer ear usually are not, but the ear is likely to be itchy, and pulling it increases the pain.

Reflexology treatment
Use reflexology in conjunction with other strategies and remedies to provide some relief from pain. Since most earaches are viral, and do not respond to antibiotics, make intensive use of complementary therapies. If pain persists, however, seek reassessment from your doctor.

**Self-help:
working your own hands
*for earache, work***
1 The ear reflex (*see p. 33*)
for tinnitus, work 1 plus
2 The sinuses (*see p. 32*)
3 The neck (*see p. 33*)

1 Work the ear
Use your left hand to support the right foot. With your right thumb, make small rotating clockwise movements on the ear reflex under the first bend of the third toe. Repeat on the left foot.

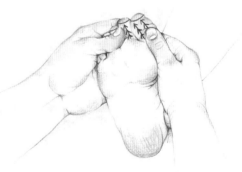

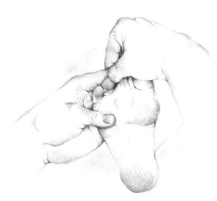

2 Work the sinuses
Support the right foot with your left hand. Use your right thumb to work up all the toes with small creeping movements, starting at the base of the big toe. Make sure you cover the entire surface of each toe.

When you reach the little toe, change hands and use your left thumb to work back across to the big toe. Repeat on the left foot.

Relaxing tactics for tinnitus

The precise cause of tinnitus, or constant ringing or buzzing in the ears, is not yet known. The latest theory is that the normal mechanism responsible for filtering out unwanted sound breaks down. It is a difficult condition to treat, though psychotherapy, to help with distraction from the noises, may help.

Reflexology treatment
Good results can be achieved by reducing the patient's level of stress, which may be particularly high where tinnitus is associated with a degree of deafness. Use the foot relaxation exercises described on pp. 24-25. In addition, work the ear reflex, as well as the sinus and neck areas. (See also p. 71.)

First aid for earache

Hold a well-padded hot water bottle to the ear.

◆

Pinch the nose hard and blow, to pop the ear. NB This may not work if the ear is very congested.

◆

Suck cough sweets or chew gum.

◆

Add a few drops of olbas, wintergreen, or peppermint oil to a bowl of hot water and inhale (see p. 46).

3 Work the neck
First work the sole of the foot. Support the right foot with your left hand and use your right thumb to work across the bases of the first 3 toes.
Then work the same area on the top of the foot, using your right index finger. Repeat on the left foot.

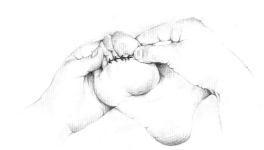

Treating eye problems
Impaired vision, conjunctivitis, styes, glaucoma

The eyes, we are told, are the windows of the soul. Not only do they reflect our inner emotional state, their own physical functioning may be affected by that inner state.

Impaired vision
Following a period of extreme overwork, a shock, or a sudden change in lifestyle, for example, people may be aware that their vision is less acute or that their eyes feel strained, painful, or oversensitive, particularly in bright sunlight. Such symptoms may appear very rapidly, even overnight. They disappear equally rapidly on release from stress.

Reflexology treatment
By relaxing the muscles of the eyes, reflexology can help ease symptoms.

Styes

Styes, boil-like eruptions on the eyelid, may be an indication of stress. General stress levels can be reduced by regular foot relaxation sessions (pp. 24-25). Support these with the practice of meditation and regular physical exercise (see Chapter Two).

Self-help:
working your own hands
for impaired vision, work

1 The eyes *(see p. 33)*

for conjunctivits or acute glaucoma, work 1 plus

2 The sinuses *(see p. 32)*

1 Work the eyes
Support the right foot with your left hand. Then place your thumb under the first bend of the the second toe. Make small rotating movements in a clockwise direction. Repeat on the left foot.

Conjunctivitis

Conjunctivitis, an inflammation of the conjunctiva (the transparent membrane covering the white of the eye and lining the lids), may give rise to swelling, soreness, and discharge. It may be caused by a simple irritation, by an allergy (more usual in adults), or by infection (common in children). It may also follow a heavy cold or an attack of sinusitis.

Reflexology treatment
Recovery may be speeded by treating the sinus areas, concentrating the work on the second toe, where the reflex point for the eye is found (see opposite).

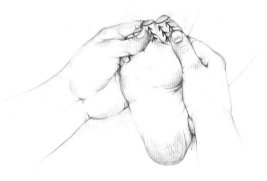

Glaucoma

Reflexology can help reduce the pain of acute glaucoma, a condition in which fluid behind the eyes increases, causing extreme pressure. Treatments help reduce this pressure. Chronic glaucoma is painless and hard to detect. Once diagnosed, daily reflexology treatments may prove helpful. Treat as for conjunctivitis.

2 Work the sinuses

Support the right foot with your left hand. Use your right thumb to work up all the toes with a small creeping movement, starting at the base of the big toe. Make sure you cover the entire surface of each toe. When you reach the little toe, change hands and use your left thumb to work back across to the big toe. Repeat on the left foot.

Support Strategies

For eyestrain, put 2 used Indian or camomile teabags in the refrigerator. When they are cold, place them on the eyes and relax. Alternatively, lie down with cool cucumber slices on your eyelids.

For styes, a warm spoon cupped over the affected eye may help bring the stye to a head. Do not attempt to burst it yourself.

For conjunctivitis, make an infusion with a camomile teabag, allowing it to stand for 10 minutes in boiling water. When it has cooled down, use it as an eye bath twice a day until the condition has cleared. Diluted witch-hazel can be used in the same way.

Treating nasal problems

Blocked or streaming nose, rhinitis, sinusitis

It has been suggested that a streaming nose and eyes are tears that have been left unshed and that a heavy cold or allergic reaction is Nature's way of getting rid of them. Whether or not you subscribe to this theory, it is worth noting the next time that you develop a heavy cold, or when an allergy goes haywire, whether it happens immediately after a difficult period, when you bottled up your feelings.

   You may already have noticed, with monotonous regularity, that your kids start getting colds as soon as they return to school after the long summer vacation. Little ones get them when they first start school – probably more to do with exposure to unfamiliar viruses than grief at leaving their mother.

Self-help:
working your own hands
for allergic reactions
(see pp. 116-117)
for sinusitis, work
1 The sinuses (*see p. 32*)
2 The eyes and ears (*see p. 33*)
3 The face (*see p. 34*)

Blocked or streaming nose

Rhinitis, inflammation of the nasal tissues, may either be caused by an infection or by an allergy. Blocked or streaming noses associated with allergic rhinitis, catarrh, or hay fever can certainly be relieved through reflexology. The aim is to strengthen the digestive system, to improve the functioning of the immune system, and to restore balance and harmony to the body so that it ceases to overreact. The treatment is as for allergies, see pp. 116-117.

1 Work the sinuses
With your left hand, support the right foot. Use your right thumb to work over the entire surface of all the toes, starting on the inside edge with the big toe. When you reach the little toe, change the support hand and use your left thumb to work back across to the big toe. Repeat on the left foot.

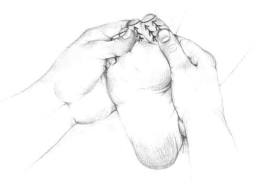

Sinusitis

The membrane lining the sinuses in the face may become inflamed, usually due to a viral infection, and in many people this often happens after a cold. A stuffy nose, painful throbbing in the affected area, and loss of the sense of smell are common symptoms.

Reflexology treatment
The aim of the treatment is to reduce inflammation. Begin by working the sinuses (p. 80), then work other areas of the face.

ear

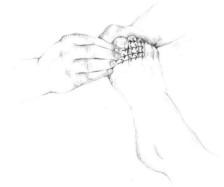

2 Work the eyes and ears
Support the right foot with your left hand. Rotate your right thumb gently on the first bends of the second and third toes. Repeat on the left foot.

3 Work the face
Make a fist with your left hand and push it into the sole of the right foot. Use your right index finger to work the areas on the front of the first 3 toes. Work across each toe, starting beneath the nail and ending where it joins the foot. Repeat on the left foot.

Support strategies

Hydrotherapy may give some relief in the case of catarrh or sinusitis. Try alternating hot and cold compresses on the forehead and on the base of the skull.

Wintergreen or peppermint oil *can be diluted and applied to the sinus area 4 times a day. Alternatively, add 2 drops of the oil to a bowl of hot water and inhale it. Do this 3 times a day.*

Do not eat *mucus-forming foods such as dairy products, sugar, and refined carbohydrates.*

Treating problems in the mouth
Toothache, mouth ulcers

Pain relief for toothache
The cause of toothache should be identified and
treated by a dentist. If a visit to the dentist is
impossible, reflexology may give short-term relief.

Reflexology treatment
Begin by working the teeth reflex points on the front
of the first three toes of each foot. You will probably
find sensitive areas just below the toe nails. For pain
relief, work the pituitary reflexes on the big toes, to
encourage the release of endorphins, the body's own
natural painkillers.

**Self-help:
working your own hands**
1 Work the teeth *(see p. 34)*

2 The pituitary *(see p. 34)*

1 Work the teeth
*Make a fist with your left hand and
push it into the sole of the right foot.
With the right index finger, work
across the fronts of the first 3 toes,
from just below the nail down to the
base. Repeat on the left foot.*

2 Work the pituitary
*Support the right foot with your
left hand. With your right thumb,
work the inside edge of the flat of
the big toe. Repeat on the left foot.*

A clove compress
*Soak a wad of cotton wool in
oil of cloves (obtainable from
the pharmacist) and place this
directly over the aching tooth.
If you cannot get hold of the
oil, use a clove instead.*

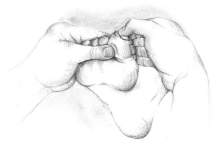

Treating mouth ulcers and their causes

Under the tongue, and on the inside of the lip or the cheek, are the usual sites of painful ulcers that may occur singly or in groups. There are a number of theories about their cause, but stress and allergies, as well as minor mouth injuries (perhaps caused by a toothbrush), may be implicated. It has also been suggested, however, that sometimes mouth ulcers are connected to digestive problems.

Reflexology treatment

If the ulcers appear to be related to stress, a course of relaxing reflexology treatments might help reduce their frequency. Follow the exercises on pp. 24-25. If an allergy is suspected, consult pp. 116-117. In the case of digestive upsets, the aim of treatment is to restore balance particularly to the stomach area, as described below.

Mouthwashes
to alleviate the pain of ulcers

Apple cider vinegar
Mix one tablespoon of the vinegar with a large tumbler full of warm water and rinse your mouth with this solution several times a day.

Tea tree oil
mouthwashes are also effective. The oil must be well diluted. Follow the instructions on the container.

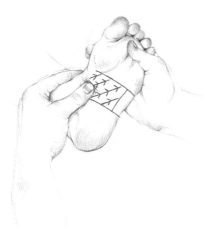

Work the stomach and pancreas
Support the left foot with the right hand. Use your left thumb, working from the inner to the outer side of the foot in the direction of the arrows. Change the supporting hand and use your right thumb to work back across the same area from the outer to the inner side of the foot. NB These reflexes are only on the left foot. (For self-help on the hands, see p. 37.)

Treating sore throats
Tonsillitis, laryngitis (hoarse, sore throat)

Inflamed tonsils make swallowing very painful, as does a sore throat. When the larynx becomes inflamed, in laryngitis, you lose your voice. In both cases the inflammation is usually caused by a viral infection and for many people these problems are the usual concomitant of having a cold.

Some mild throat problems may be due to an irritant, such as paint or cigarette fumes. Laryngitis may also result from misuse of the voice, as amateur actors or singers often find to their cost.

Reflexology treatment
The treatment is effective in easing pain. In addition to the throat and sinus reflexes, work the cervical spine to increase the blood supply to the throat and to ease congestion. Then work the spleen to build up immunity and resistance to infection.

Self-help:
working your own hands
1 The throat *(see p. 33)*
2 The sinuses *(see p. 32)*
3 The cervical spine *(see p. 34)*
4 The spleen *(see p. 31)*

1 Work the throat
With the left hand, support the right foot. Use your right index finger to work the area on the inside edge of the big toe, where it joins the foot. The area is small, but you can often locate it precisely because of its sensitivity. Treat it by pressing in and making small clockwise rotations. Repeat on the left foot.

throat area

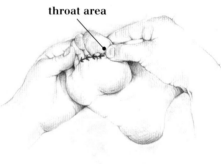

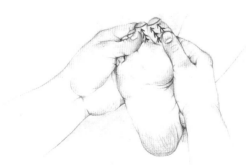

2 Work the sinuses
Support the right foot with your left hand. Use your right thumb to work up the toes with a small creeping movement, starting at the base of the big toe. Make sure you cover the entire surface of each toe. When you reach the little toe, change hands and use your left thumb to work back across to the big toe.

Repeat on the left foot, again changing hands to work back from the little toe.

Support Strategies

Drink a lot *Lemon and honey or herbal teas or fruit juices are good. Avoid mucus-forming milky drinks.*

Eat less *If you have a temperature, don't eat at all. Let the vital healing energy of the body deal with the infection. When the temperature drops, take light meals again.*

To lower a temperature, *soak a towel in cold water, wring it out, and cover both feet with it. This old-fashioned remedy redirects heat from the head to warm up the feet.*

Step up your vitamins *Vitamin C: 1g 3 times a day; vitamin B complex: high dose, 1 daily*

Onion and honey *To ease laryngitis, boil an onion in just enough water to cover it. Strain off the liquid and dissolve 1 teaspoon of honey in it. Take 3 teaspoons of the mixture every 3 hours.*

Cider vinegar gargle *For sore throats in general, gargle with 2 teaspoonsful of apple cider vinegar to a cup of warm water.*

Diet *If you get regular infections, eat lots of fresh fruit and vegetables, little or no sugar, more garlic and onions.*

3 Work the cervical spine
With your left hand, support the top of the right foot. Use your right thumb to work the spine reflex points on the inside of the foot, concentrating particularly on the cervical spine area on the inside edge of the big toe. Repeat on the left foot.

4 Work the spleen
With your right hand, support the left foot. With your left thumb, work out the oblong area indicated between the diaphragm and waist lines. Start on the inside edge and work across the area and back. (Left foot only.)

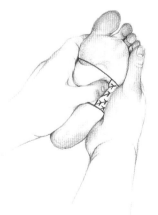

Problems in the chest area: 1

Angina

The success of any long-term treatment for angina depends on a change in lifestyle to prevent the condition becoming worse. Characterized by a pressing, gripping, continuous tight pain in the middle of the chest , possibly extending up into the arms, back, neck, or jaw, it is caused by insufficient oxygen reaching the heart muscle. It is often brought on by overexertion, emotional upheaval, smoking, or even just by eating a heavy meal. The only immediate treatment is rest.

Reflexology treatment
Angina responds well to reflexology, which helps reduce stress levels, improves nerve and muscle function, and increases the blood supply to the heart. The main areas to work are those of the heart, lung, and ribcage. If you have time, work the liver (p. 29) and upper part of the spine (p. 27) as well.

Allow the patient to relax for 15 minutes or so before treatment, perhaps with a guided visualization (see p. 45) during a foot relaxation (pp. 24-25). Then work for 15 minutes on each foot.

**Self-help:
working your own hands**
1 The heart *(see p. 37)*
2 The lungs *(see p. 32)*

Angina alert!
Angina pains that continue in spite of rest, cause paleness, sweating, or collapse may not be angina but a heart attack. This is a medical emergency.

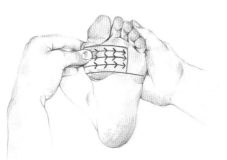

1 Work the heart
NB The heart reflex is only found on the left foot. Do not overwork it!
Support the top of the left foot with your right hand. Use your left thumb to work the area in the direction shown. Do this 2 or 3 times, no more.

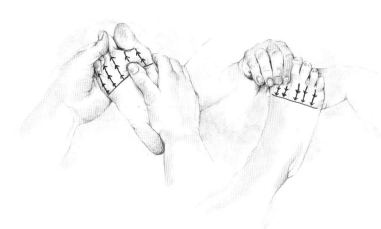

2 Work the lungs

First work the sole of the foot. Support the right foot with your left hand. Use your right thumb to work from the base of the diaphragm line up to where the toes join the foot. Work this reflex 2 or 3 times.

Next work the top of the right foot. Make a fist with your left hand and press it into the sole of the foot, to open up the grooves on the top. Use your right index finger to work down these grooves. Work this reflex 2 or 3 times. Repeat on the left foot

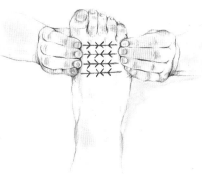

3 Relax the ribcage

Press both thumbs into the sole of the right foot. Use the fingers of both hands to creep across the top of the foot until they meet in the middle. Repeat on the left foot.

Support Strategies

Give up smoking!

Review your diet See p. 41.

Reduce your alcohol intake, and don't binge!

Take brisk exercise daily! Walking and swimming are both good. Exercise till you can feel your heart beating faster and you gently perspire, but do not overexert yourself. Gradually increase the time spent.

Yoga is good exercise, de-stressing and energetically healing (see pp. 43-44).

Relaxation Try to spend at least 15 minutes each day relaxing (see p. 42). A good time to do this is after exercising.

Avoid stress-inducing situations. Or learn, through counselling or psychotherapy, to handle them more appropriately.

Problems in the chest area: 2

Asthma

Children, particularly those who live in cities, are suffering in increasing numbers from asthma, and seem to respond especially well to reflexology. Start a treatment, whether for child or adult, after some breathing exercises (p. 42), which should help to relax the patient. Follow these with the diaphragm relaxation exercise (p. 24). Then work the areas of the heart, lung, and thoracic spine to improve lung function and relax the shoulders and ribcage. Many asthmatic people have taut neck and shoulder muscles through "hunching" up during attacks.

If the asthma is an allergic reaction, consult pp. 116-117 for advice on coping with allergies.

Asthma can be life threatening and these strategies are not intended to take the place of the treatment prescribed by your doctor; they are meant to support that treatment, perhaps eventually leading to less need for medication or helping to control a flare up.

**Self-help:
working your own hands**
1 The heart *(see p. 37)*

2 The lungs *(see p. 32)*

3 The spine *(see p. 34)*

1 Relax the diaphragm
Support the right foot with your left hand, as shown. Edge the right thumb a little further along the diaphragm line (where the foot changes colour), each time you bring the toes down over the left thumb, in a back and forth rocking motion.

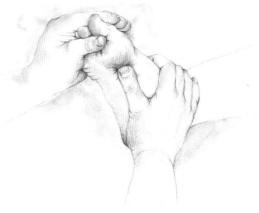

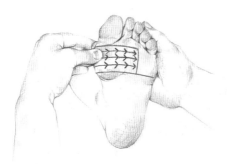

2 Work the heart
Support the top of the left foot with your right hand. Use your left thumb to work the area in the direction shown. Do this 2 or 3 times, no more. You must not overwork this area. (NB The heart reflex is only found on the left foot.)

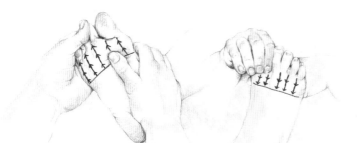

3 Work the lungs

First work the sole of the foot. Support the right foot with your left hand. Use your right thumb to work up each area from the diaphragm line to the base of each toe. Work this reflex 2 or 3 times.

Next work the top of the right foot. Make a fist with your left hand and press it into the sole of the foot, to open up the grooves on the top. Use your right index finger to work down these grooves. Work this reflex 2 or 3 times.

Repeat on the left foot.

4 Work the thoracic spine

With your left hand, support the right foot. Use your right thumb to work the spine, concentrating on the area between the waist line and the beginning of the cervical spine at the base of the big toe (see map, p. 17).

Repeat on the left foot.

Support Strategies

Keep on the move. *Swimming – particularly breaststroke – is excellent exercise for the respiratory system. If you are susceptible to pollen or dust you are less likely to encounter them in the swimming pool than on the playing field.*

Make deep relaxed breathing *exercises part of your daily routine (see p. 42).*

Keep *your weight down.*

Cut out *mucus-forming foods (see p. 81).*

Vacuum clean *your home, particularly your bedroom, regularly and wipe all surfaces with a damp cloth at least once a week. It is essential to keep your environment as dust free as possible.*

Strong coffee *helps in an asthma attack, especially if you are not in the habit of drinking it strong.*

Problems in the chest area: 3

Bronchitis, mastitis

Smoking is the main cause of chronic bronchitis, though a polluted atmosphere is also a major contributory factor. Coughing, wheezing, and breathlessness are symptoms of this disease in which the airways in the lungs become narrower and obstructed. Acute bronchitis, the result of a bacterial or viral infection, develops suddenly but usually clears after a few days. The very young as well as elderly people and, of course, smokers are all particularly vulnerable, especially during the winter.

Reflexology treatment
Follow the treatment for asthma on pp. 88-89. Treat the digestive system (pp. 100-101), as well, since a weakness in the digestive system may cause excess mucus. To help build up resistance, treat the spleen as described below.

Work the spleen
With the right hand, support the top of the left foot. With your left thumb, work the oblong area between the diaphragm and the waist line. Start on the inside edge and work in the direction shown. Then.work back. (Left foot only.)

**Self-help:
working your own hands
*for bronchitis, work***

1 As for asthma *(see p. 88)*

2 The digestive system
(see pp. 35-37)

3 The spleen *(see p. 37)*

for mastitis, work

The breast *(see p. 32)*

Support Strategies

Daily deep breathing *exercises (as described on p. 42) expand lung capacity. Older people may prefer to practise them lying on a bed rather than on the floor. Those with bad bronchitis may need to do them sitting in an upright chair.*

Stop smoking/don't start!

Vitamin C *in large doses helps protect against viruses. A 1g-slow-release tablet daily should be enough. Increase to 1g 3 times a day if you get a cold.*

Wintergreen, juniper, *and eucalyptus oils give off soothing aromas that help ease breathing. Put a few drops in an electric vaporizer and keep it in the bedroom overnight (see p. 47).*

Mastitis

This condition, in which inflammation of the glands makes the breasts swollen and lumpy, affects many women, and usually lasts for several days before their period starts. It often coincides with PMT or PMS, which is discussed on pp. 104-107.

Reflexology treatment

Reflexology can ease the pain and discomfort of mastitis by helping to balance hormonal secretions and relieve congested ducts.

Work on the endocrine system which deals with hormonal responses throughout the body. (See the complete treatment for the endocrine system on pp. 108-109.) Then work out the area to the breast, which shares its reflex points with the lung, but is contacted mainly on the top of the foot.

Support Strategies

Evening primrose oil *Take 6-8 capsules daily and be prepared to wait for 3 months before they have any effect.*

Make sure your bra *fits well and wear it all the time during PMT lumps or breast tenderness.*

Get to know your breasts. *Learn how to examine your breasts. Then check them once a month, after your period. Breast cancer is most often found on self-examination. Lumpy breasts do not make you more prone to breast cancer, but do make it harder to detect. Seek medical advice immediately if you discover anything that is different from usual.*

Work the breast

First work the sole of the right foot, supporting the foot with your left hand. Use your right thumb to work from the diaphragm line on the inside edge of the foot, moving in straight lines up to the bases of the toes. Next make a fist with your left hand and press it into the sole of the foot. Use your right index finger to work down the grooves on the top of the foot. Repeat these steps on the left foot. For self help on the hands, see p. 32.

Problems in the chest area: 4

Palpitations

The old enemy, stress, is the most common precipitating factor for palpitations, an awareness of the heart beating at a different rate or rhythm than usual. If you suspect that stress is the cause, consult Chapter Five, where you will find advice on how to make stress manageable. Other likely causes are excessive intakes of alcohol or caffeine, or food allergies.

Palpitations may, however, be symptomatic of a heart condition. If you feel ill with them or if you experience a very rapid heartbeat, like a "bird fluttering" in the chest, seek medical advice immediately. In any event, consult your doctor if palpitations persist.

Reflexology treatment
A reflexology treatment that induces relaxation and helps balance the patient's chi, or vital energy, covers the heart, spine (the nerve centre of the entire body), and the solar plexus reflexes.

Begin by going through all the relaxation exercises (pp.24–25) and give the treatment daily while palpitations continue.

**Self-help:
working your own hands**
1 The heart (*see p. 37*)
2 The spine (*see p. 34*)
3 The solar plexus, behind the stomach (*see p. 37*)

The heart centre
Our heart centres are like the sun, radiating warmth and light when we are happy or in love. Negative, painful thoughts are clouds that cross the heart. If feelings of fear, anger, or jealousy have invaded your heart like black storm clouds, try, while having your reflexology treatment, to visualize them surrounded by a golden light and feel them melt away.

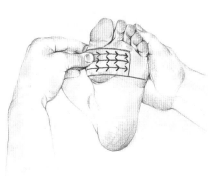

1 Work the heart
The heart reflex is found only on the left foot. Do not overwork it. With your right hand, support the top of the left foot. Use your left thumb to work the area shown, a maximum of 3 times.

2 Relax the diaphragm

Place your left thumb beneath the toes on the right foot as shown. Bring the toes down over the thumb, moving the right thumb a little farther along the diaphragm line each time you do so setting up a steady rhythm as the toes rock to and fro.

Repeat on the left foot.

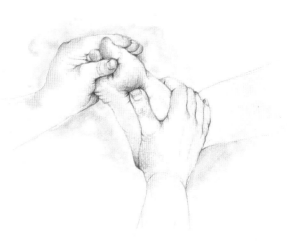

3 Work the spine

With your left hand, support the right foot. Use your right thumb to work up the spinal reflex points.

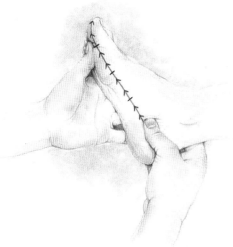

4 Work the solar plexus

On this reflex point, you work with the patient's breath, so explain to them what you want them to do before you begin

Hold the left foot with your right hand. Place your left thumb on the solar plexus reflex and ask the patient to breathe in as you apply deep pressure on this point. Release the pressure as he or she exhales. Do this for 3 or 4 minutes at a time.

This treatment often produces wonderfully quick results, inducing deep relaxation, even sleepiness. At the same time, however, treating the solar plexus often releases deep seated feelings and tensions, so neither you nor your patient should be dismayed by an emotional reaction to work on this area.

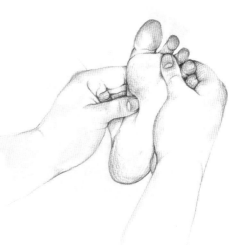

Treating back problems
Lumbago, sciatica

Relieving lumbago and other back pains

Osteopaths say you are as old as your spine, and most people who have suffered with back pain will agree that it makes them feel much older as well as miserable. Poor posture and lack of exercise are contributory factors. Structure governs function: using cars and elevators, rather than walking, leads to weak abdominal muscles, which fail to give enough support to the upper back.

Reflexology treatment

For relief of lumbago and other back pains, you can safely work the skeletal system (as shown below) 12 or 14 times in one session. If the pain is acute, do this 3 or 4 times a day, if possible, until the condition improves.

**Self-help:
working your own hands
*for lumbago, work***
1 The coccyx (*see p. 33*)
2 The hip/pelvis (*see p. 33*)
3 The spine (*see p. 34*)
for sciatica, work 1, 2, 3 plus
4 The sciatic nerve
(*see map, p. 19*)

1 Work the coccyx
With your right hand, hold the right foot away from the body. Use the 4 left fingers to work the area shown. Repeat on the left foot.

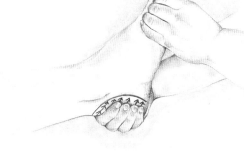

2 Work the hip/pelvis
Hold the right foot away from the body with your left hand. With the 4 right fingers, work the area shown on the outside edge of the foot. Repeat on the left foot.

Sciatica

The cause of this searing pain down the leg is compression of the nerves that make up the sciatic nerve, the largest nerve in the body. The commonest cause of this is spasm in the surrounding muscles. This may be triggered by a misalignment of the joints in the lower spine, by osteoarthritis, or, sometimes, by a disc problem.

Reflexology treatment
Follow the treatment recommended for lumbago, which helps by improving the blood supply to the affected area. And since reflexology acts well in reducing extreme pain, also work on the brain area to encourage the release of endorphins, the natural "feel good" chemicals that help block pain.

Look after your back

Sleep on a firm, young mattress (not more than 10 years old).

◆

Your pillow should support your head in the same position as when you are standing.

◆

Sit in an upright chair and do not slump. Roll a towel and use it to support your lower back.

◆

Ensure your desk/chair height is correct for your own height.

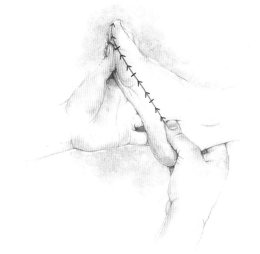

3 Work the spine
Support the right foot with your left hand. Use your right thumb to work the spine reflexes along the inside edge of the foot. Repeat on the left foot.

4 Work the sciatic nerve
Support the right foot with the right hand. Place your left index finger just behind the ankle bone and work in a line up the leg for about 10cm (4in). Repeat on the left foot.

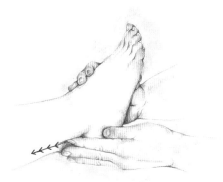

Treating the arms & hands: 1

Stiff shoulder, tennis elbow

Loosening a stiff shoulder

Overuse of the shoulder joint, lifting heavy objects, or an arthritic condition may all cause the shoulder to become stiff and painful. Uncomfortable as it may be, it is important to keep the shoulder moving: swinging it very gently from side to side, raising it as far as possible to the front and then taking it backward will help prevent its becoming progressively stiffer.

Reflexology treatment

Work out the entire shoulder and neck area, on both feet. If the problem shoulder is on the right, you will probably find sensitivity in the shoulder reflex on the right foot. For the sake of balance, however, it is necessary to treat the shoulder reflexes on both left and right feet. Use the same treatment for any sports injury that has affected the shoulders.

**Self-help:
working your own hands
*for a stiff shoulder, work***

1 The shoulder (*see p. 34*)

2 The cervical spine (*see p. 34*)

for tennis elbow, work 1, 2 &

3 The elbow (*see p. 35*)

1 Work the shoulder

To treat the right shoulder, support the right foot with your left hand. With your right thumb, work the area below the little toe in the direction shown. Change hands and work back across the area with your left thumb. Then treat the shoulder area on the left foot.

Frozen peas

Ice packs are good for all joint, tendon, or muscle pains. Use a bag of frozen peas (or frozen corn) applying it to the affected area for 15 minutes on, then 15 minutes off.

Tennis elbow: reducing inflammation

This condition does not – despite its name – simply arise from over-exertion on the tennis court. Excessive use of the forearm, muscular strain caused by lifting, or by carrying a heavy weight, may cause the tendon that attaches the overused muscle to the arm to become inflamed. This causes pain on the outer side of the elbow, below the joint.

Keep the joint moving, gently, through the full possible range of movement.

Reflexology treatment

Reflexology can come to the rescue in relieving pain, settling down the inflammation in the tendon, as an improvement in nerve and blood supply occurs, and normalizing the functioning of the arm and elbow. Work out the areas to the cervical spine and elbow.

Shouldering burdens

Use a back-pack arrangement whenever possible. Even a light bag slung over the shoulder causes hunching, which becomes a habit and leads to problems.

When carrying heavy shopping or a young child, distribute the weight evenly between the arms. Habitually using the same arm to bear heavy weights not only causes stress to the arm but, because of the imbalance, will almost inevitably lead to hip and lower back problems.

2 Work the cervical spine

With your left hand, support the top of the right foot. Use your right thumb to work the spine reflexes on the inside of the foot, concentrating particularly on the area on the inside edge of the big toe. Repeat on the left foot.

3 Work the elbow

To treat the right elbow, support the right foot with your right hand. Use your left index and middle fingers to work the triangular elbow area on the outside edge of the foot. To treat the left elbow, work the elbow area on the left foot. Treat both feet.

Treating the arms & hands: 2
Carpal tunnel syndrome, Raynaud's syndrome, R.S.I.

Pain relief for carpal tunnel syndrome

This problem is very common in women and is often triggered by the hormonal changes in pregnancy and the menopause. People who perform repetitive tasks with their hands, such as typists, are particularly susceptible, but it may also follow trauma to the wrist. Caused by compression of the median nerve as it passes between the bones and ligaments of the wrist, carpal tunnel syndrome leads to pain and weakness when gripping, and tingling, aching, or a feeling of "deadness," which is usually worse at night.

Reflexology treatment

Working the cervical spine offers some relief, since nerves from this area supply impulses to the shoulders, arms, elbows, and wrists. After this, work the elbow, to further help circulation to the hand. Working directly on the area of stress is also beneficial. Treatments should be given daily.

**Self-help:
working your own hands
*for carpal tunnel syndrome,
work***

1 The cervical spine *(see p. 34)*

2 The elbow *(see p. 35)*

for Raynaud's syndrome, work

1 The heart *(see p. 37)*

2 The lung *(see p. 32)*

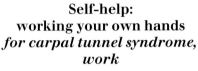

1 Work the cervical spine
Supporting the right foot with your left hand, use your right thumb to work up the spine, concentrating on the area on the inside edge of the big toe. (See map, p. 17.) Repeat on the left foot. Then do the ankle-freeing exercise (see p. 24).

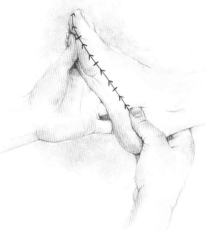

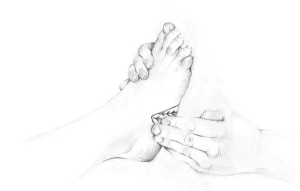

2 Work the elbow
To treat the right elbow, support the right foot at the top with your right hand. Use your left index and middle fingers to work the triangular elbow area on the outside edge of the foot.

Raynaud's syndrome: improving circulation

This circulatory problem means that because the capillaries contract very easily, the extremities – fingers and toes – are starved of blood and become white and numb. It is usually triggered by cold weather.

When these symptoms arise from another underlying disorder, it is called Raynaud's syndrome or phenomenon. This is much commoner than Raynaud's disease, for which the same symptoms have no known cause.

Reflexology treatment
The aim of treatment is to improve the circulation by working the heart and lungs. Do this for 15 minutes.

Repetitive strain injury (R.S.I.)

Long periods each day manipulating a computer mouse or a keyboard may lead to severe pain that radiates from the fingers to the shoulder. It is essential to take steps to prevent the condition becoming incapacitating. Seek professional advice on how to minimize the risks, and, if necessary, take a long break from your machine.

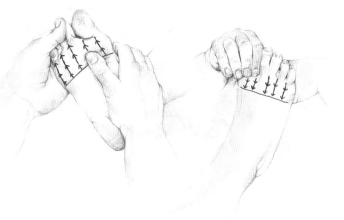

1 Work the heart

NB The heart reflex is only found on the left foot. Do not overwork it.
Support the top of the left foot with your right hand. Use your left thumb to work the area in the direction shown. Do this a maximum of 3 times.

2 Work the lungs

Support the right foot with your left hand and work the area indicated on the sole of the foot. Then, press your left fist into the sole, to open the grooves on the top. Work down these grooves with your right index finger. Repeat on the left foot.

Key system 1:
The digestive system

Reflexology is particularly successful in treating many common ailments related to the digestive system. Some of these may be caused principally by food intake, others may also include a strong stress component: problems, such as irritable bowel syndrome and colitis, for example, are common in individuals who are prone to stress. Treating the digestive system in order to improve its functioning also produces good results where a weakness in this area is thought to play a part in allergic reactions.

Always treat the entire system, as described here. Where stress is suspected as a contributory factor, start by relaxing the feet (see pp. 24-25).

Self-help:
working your own hands
1 The liver and gallbladder
(see p. 35)
2 The stomach, pancreas,
and spleen *(see p. 37)*
3 The intestinal area *(see p. 35)*

1 Work the liver and gallbladder
Support the right foot with your left hand. Use your right thumb to work from the inside to the outside edge of the foot, between the waist and diaphragm lines.

Then work back over the same area in the opposite direction. Do this with your left thumb, supporting the foot with your right hand.

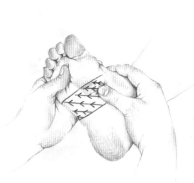

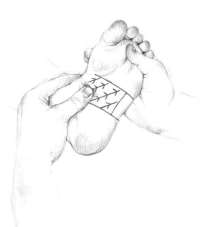

2 Work the stomach and pancreas
Support the left foot with your right hand. Use your left thumb to work from the inside to the outside edge of the foot over the area indicated. Change the support hand and work back over the same area in the opposite direction, from the outside to the inside edge.

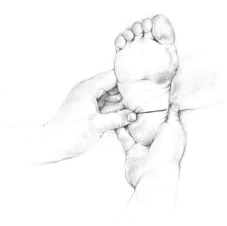

3 Work the ileocecal valve

Use your right hand to support the heel of the right foot. Place your left thumb on the heel line and work the reflex point with the "hooking out" technique described on p. 29. (Right foot only.)

4 Work the ascending and transverse colon, and small intestine

With your left hand, support the right foot. Use your right thumb to work the area between the waist line and the pelvic line. Work across from the inside to the outside edge.

Change the support hand and use your left thumb to work back across the same area, from the outside to the inside edge.

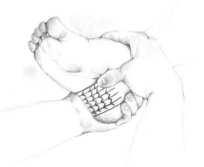

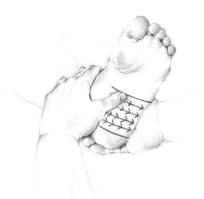

5 Work the transverse, descending, and sigmoid colon, and small intestine

Use your right hand to support the heel of the left foot. With your left thumb, work the area from the waist line down to the midway point between the pelvic line and the base of the heel. Do this first from the inside to the outside edge.

Change the support hand and use your right thumb to work the same area from the outside to the inside edge.

Treating digestive problems
Gallstones, IBS, and other common ailments

Intensive treatment for gallstones

The classic candidate for gallstones is said to be female, fair, fat, and forty. After the age of about 70, men and women are affected equally.

Gallstones occur when a component of bile (produced by the gallbladder) becomes supersaturated and starts to form stones. The stones only become a problem if they get stuck in the bile duct. If they are not causing symptoms, they are not removed.

Reflexology treatment

Some people who have had reflexology while awaiting surgery eventually find that an operation is unnecessary because the symptoms have gone. It is not possible to attribute this conclusively to the treatment. It means, however, that the stones are no longer in the bile duct, though there may still be some in the gallbladder.

In any event, reflexology can be of assistance in treating the discomfort of gallstones. The most important area to work is the liver (p. 100). You will probably find acute sensitivity here, so only use the amount of pressure that is acceptable to the patient. Work over the area 2 or 3 times, repeating this procedure twice a day until the sensitivity decreases.

Self-help:
working your own hands
Work the liver and gallbladder
(see p. 35)

Support Strategies
Gallstones

Keep your weight down!

*A **high-fibre diet** is recommended. Cut out sugar and refined foods. Eat less animal fat.*

***Herbal remedies** are said to be effective in treating gallstones. Seek the advice of a professional herbalist, though; do not attempt to treat yourself.*

If you suffer from indigestion...

***Camomile/peppermint teas** are good for the digestion. Drink them at any time, but not for at least half an hour after eating. Do not drink any liquid with meals, since it makes digestion harder.*

***Rosemary**, in an infusion, calms the nerves and aids digestion. Take 1 cup 3 times a day.*

***Arrowroot** settles the stomach. Combine 1 tablespoon with enough water to make a smooth paste. Bring the mixture to the boil and mix it with a little warm milk. Or take slippery elm food in the same way.*

Taking the stress out of IBS

Irritable bowel syndrome (IBS) produces a wide range of symptoms, including intermittent abdominal pain, bouts of diarrhea, nausea, constipation, indigestion, bloating, and flatulence, as well as headaches. People suffering from it also seem to suffer from higher than average levels of anxiety.

Though the causes of IBS are not clear, it seems to be associated in some instances with a food allergy.

Reflexology treatment

The dual goal of treatment is to improve the function of the bowel and to help combat stress. The relaxing influence of treatments helps by calming the overstimulated digestive areas and bringing the body back into balance.

Begin with the general foot relaxation session (pp. 24-25). Then treat the digestive system (see pp. 100-101). Work for at least 10 minutes on each foot, daily if possible. Patients who are constipated may have a bowel action within an hour or so of treatment.

(pp. 24-25). Then treat the digestive system (see pp. 100-101).

Support Strategies
IBS

Regular excercise not only helps reduce stress, it also helps the functioning of the digestive system.

The Top 4 IBS-causing culprits are:1 Wheat 2 Yeast (bread, cheese, alcohol) 3 Sugar 4 Dairy products. To find out if any of these is at the root of your problem, keep an allergy diary (see p. 116).

(see p. 116).

Ban bran from your diet for a while: it makes many IBS sufferers worse. Stopping wheat, or only eating spelt or white flour, may solve the problem.

Acidophilus helps restore normal gut flora, often unbalanced in chronic cases of IBS. It is readily available in commercial yogurts.

If you suffer from constipation or diarrhea...

A high-fibre diet, with lots of raw vegetables, wholemeal bread, and jacket potatoes, should encourage normal bowel function. However, people suffering from diarrhea should avoid loosening foods such as dried fruits.

Don't substitute bread for roughage (fruit and vegetables) if you are prone to diarrhea. Not only are fruit and vegetables very health protective, bread is more likely to be the prime dietary trigger of your problem.

Problems with periods: 1
Painful periods

Though painful periods can affect women of all ages, young teenage girls seem to be particularly susceptible. The abdominal cramps caused by muscular spasms of the uterine wall, or of the strong muscular walls of the pelvic cavity, vary in intensity but may be incapacitating.

Reflexology treatment
Considerable relief from period pains can be achieved by working not only the reproductive reflexes but also the lumbar spine, in order to stimulate the nerve and blood supply to the pelvic area. Remember that constipation exacerbates pelvic pain, so if you suspect that this could be a factor, work out the intestinal areas as shown in working the digestive system on pp. 100-101.

Self-help:
working your own hands
1 The uterus (*see p. 36*)
2 The fallopian tubes (*see p. 37*)
3 The ovaries (*see p. 36*)
4 The lumbar spine (*see p. 34*)
5 The intestines (*see p. 35*)

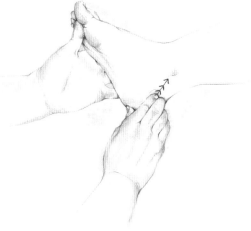

1 Work the uterus
Support the right foot with your left hand. Use the right index finger to work in a straight line from the base of the heel to the ankle bone.
    Repeat on the left foot.

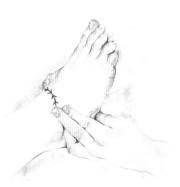

2 Work the fallopian tubes
Start on the right foot. While pressing both thumbs into the sole of the foot, work the index and middle fingers of both hands toward each other over the top of the foot. Repeat on the left foot.

3 Work the ovaries

With the right hand, support the right foot, tilting it outward, to relax the muscles and ligaments in the ankle. Use your left index finger to work the area shown. Switch hands and work the same area on the left foot.

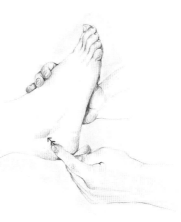

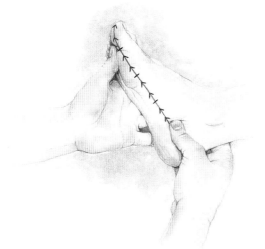

4 Work the lumbar spine

Hold the right foot away from the body with your left hand. With your right thumb, work the spine reflexes on the inside edge of the foot, concentrating particularly on the area between the pelvic line and the waist line (see map, p. 17). Repeat on the left foot.

After working the spine, use the ankle-freeing exercise (see p. 24).

Support Strategies

Calming camomile tea *helps relieve nervous tension. Make a pot as soon as cramps start, and sip it throughout the day.*

Aromatherapy *Relax in a warm bath to which you have added 6 drops of Roman camomile, marjoram, or cypress oil.*

Diet *Increase your calcium intake, not by eating more dairy products, but by eating beans, lentils, chickpeas, and green leafy vegetables, such as watercress, kale, parsley, spinach, and broccoli.*

A hot water bottle *on the abdominal area or lower back helps to ease pain.*

Problems with periods: 2

Premenstrual tension (PMT)

PMT or PMS (Premenstrual Syndrome) affects certain women, particularly those in their 30s and 40s, at a regular time in their monthly cycle. Sore, swollen breasts, bloated abdomen, weight gain, headaches, backache, and distressing mood changes are just some of the more than 150 symptoms associated with it. (See also mastitis, p. 91.)

Reflexology treatment
As well as having a relaxing, stress-reducing effect, reflexology can correct hormonal imbalances (through work on the endocrine system) and help to eliminate excess body fluid (through work on the urinary and lymphatic systems). Treat daily for a fortnight before the period is due.

Self-help:
working your own hands
1 The neck/thyroid (*see p. 33*)
2 The brain (*see p. 34*)
3 The ovaries (*see p. 36*)
4 The kidneys (*see p. 36*)
5 The groin lymph (*see p. 36*)

1 Work the neck/thyroid
First work the sole of the right foot. Support the foot with your left hand and use your right thumb to work across the bases of the first 3 toes.
Now work the top of the foot (shown left), using your right index finger to work across the bases of the first 3 toes. Repeat on the left foot.

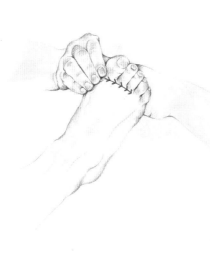

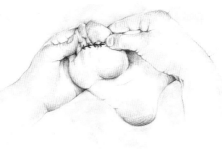

2 Work the brain

With your left hand, support the right foot. Use your right thumb to apply pressure to the tops of the first 3 toes. Repeat on the left foot.

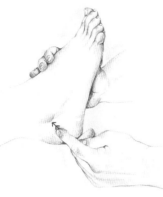

3 Work the ovaries

With the right hand, support the right foot, tilting it outward to relax the ankle. Use your left index finger to work the area shown. Repeat on the left foot.

4 Work the kidneys

Support the right foot with the left hand. Use your right thumb to apply pressure to the kidney reflex and then rotate the foot around this thumb. (This way of working causes least discomfort in this very sensitive area.) Repeat on the left foot.

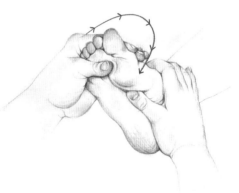

5 Work the groin lymph

This shares the same reflex as the fallopian tube. Start on the right foot. Press both thumbs into the sole of the foot. Work the index and middle fingers of each hand toward each other over the top of the foot.

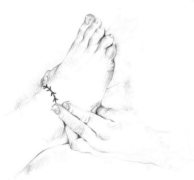

Key system 2:
The endocrine system

Hormones produced by the endocrine glands are responsible for growth, metabolism, sexual development and function, and response to stress. Any increase or decrease in the production of a hormone interferes with the process it controls. Thus hormones have a direct or indirect effect on our emotional state.

Reflexology has the effect of balancing hormone production, and is successful in treating menstrual problems and depression as well as thyroid problems (both over- and underactive). The endocrine system is highly susceptible to being thrown out of balance by emotional as well as physiological stress, so regular relaxation treatments (see pp. 24-25 and Chapter Two) should be offered in addition to work on the endocrine system.

Self-help:
working your own hands

1 The thyroid and neck *(see p. 33)*

2 The brain area *(see p. 34)*

3 The adrenals (kidney reflex) *(see p. 36)*

4 The pancreas *(see p. 37)*

5 The ovaries/testes *(see p. 36)*

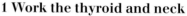

1 Work the thyroid and neck
Support the right foot with your left hand. Use your right thumb to work across the area where the first 3 toes join the foot. Do this 2 or 3 times, both on the sole (shown below) and on the top of the foot (shown left).

Repeat on the left foot.

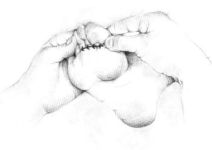

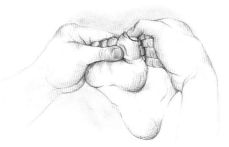

2 Work the pituitary, hypothalamus, and pineal gland

With your left hand, support the right foot. Use your right thumb to work over the top half of the big toe, on the inside edge, in the direction shown. Do this 2 or 3 times.

Repeat on the left foot.

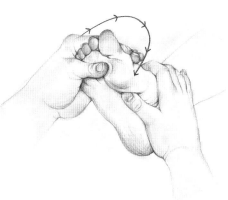

3 Work the adrenals

The adrenals lie on top of the kidneys.
Support the right foot with your left hand. With your right thumb, apply pressure to the kidney reflex point (as indicated) and rotate the foot around it.
Repeat on the left foot.

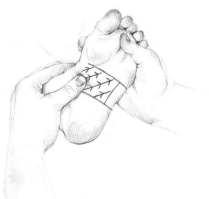

4 Work the pancreas

Support the left foot with your right hand. Use your left thumb to work from the inside to the outside edge of the foot in the direction indicated over the area shown. Change the support hand and work back over the same area in the opposite direction, from the outside to the inside edge. (Left foot only.)

5 Work the ovaries/testes

Support the right foot with your right hand, tilting the foot outward, to relax the muscles and ligaments in the ankles. Use your left index finger to work the line from the base of the heel up to the ankle bone. Do this 2 or 3 times.
Repeat on the left foot.

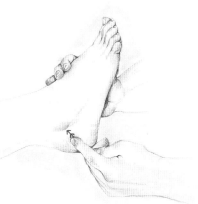

Treating bladder problems: 1
Cystitis, urinary incontinence

Reducing the distress of cystitis
One of the most common female urinary complaints, this inflammatory condition of the bladder causes frequent (often uncontrollable) and very painful urination as well as pain in the lower pelvic area.

Sexual intercourse (particularly after a long period of abstension), tight clothing (which prevents free circulation of air around the pelvic area), and vaginal douches may all cause a sensitivity in the bladder area. Not drinking enough, leading to concentrated urine, serves to exacerbate the problem.

Reflexology treatment
Reflexology can assist in reducing inflammation. During an attack, treat the urinary system for a couple of minutes on each foot several times a day. Regular treatment is effective in preventing cystitis.

Self-help:
working your own hands
for cystitis, work

1 The bladder and ureter (*see p. 35*)

2 The kidneys (*see p. 36*)

for incontinence, work 1, 2, &

3 The lumbar spine (*see p. 34*)

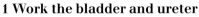

1 Work the bladder and ureter
Support the right foot with your left hand. With your right thumb, work over the soft, puffy area on the inside edge of the foot. Then work along the ureter line to the kidney. Always work on the inside edge of the ligament line. Repeat on the left foot.

2 Work the kidneys
Support the right foot with the left hand. Use your left thumb to apply pressure to the kidney reflex and then rotate the foot around the thumb. (This way of working causes least discomfort in this very sensitive area.)

Urinary incontinence

Coughing, sneezing, or lifting something heavy may prompt the involuntary leakages of urine many women experience due to stress incontinence. This problem often arises after childbirth, which causes a slackening in the muscles and ligaments of the pelvic floor that support the uterus and the vagina, the bladder, and urethra (the tube down which urine flows from the bladder). A similar slackening occurs simply with age, and elderly women, particularly, often suffer from urinary incontinence.

Reflexology treatment
Frequent reflexology treatments shortly after childbirth may help prevent stress incontinence. If the condition already has a hold, reflexology can help reduce its impact. In the case of the elderly, reflexology has proved extremely beneficial, particularly if treatments are given daily.

Support Strategies
Cystitis
Cider vinegar *Mix 2 teaspoons in a tumbler full of water, with honey, and drink 4 tumblers a day, to prevent urinary tract infections.*

Wear *cotton underwear and avoid tights.*

Do not use *vaginal talcs or deodorants.*

Incontinence
Strengthen your pelvic *floor by* ***pretending*** *to stop and start the flow of urine, but not while actually urinating. Mothers-to-be should start during pregnancy and continue after the birth.*

Elderly *people, keep moving to keep* ***all*** *your muscles toned!*

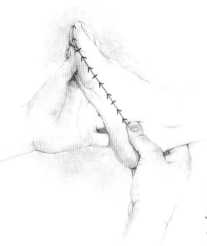

3 Work the lumbar spine
With your left hand, hold the right foot away from the body and use your right thumb to work the area between the pelvic line and the waist line on the inside edge of the foot. Repeat on the left foot.

Treating bladder problems: 2
Kidney stones (renal colic), enlarged prostate

Relieving the pain of kidney stones

The pain associated with the passing of a kidney stone is severe in the extreme. The problem seems to affect men more than women, and it occurs frequently in the summer months, perhaps due to insufficient intake of fluid at a time when the body is losing a lot through sweating.

The reason for a tendency to form stones should be established through medical investigation.

Reflexology treatment

The passing of small stones has been assisted by reflexology. After stones have been passed, one treatment a week should suffice on a "maintenance" basis, to prevent a recurrence.

**Self-help:
working your own hands
*for kidney stones, work***

1, 2 The bladder, ureter, and kidneys *(see pp. 35, 36)*

***for enlarged prostate,
work 1, 2, &***

3 The prostate gland *(see p. 36)*

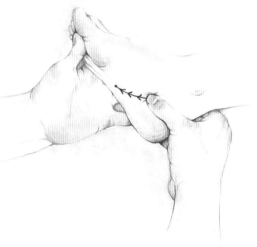

1 Work the bladder and ureter

Support the right foot with your left hand. Use your right thumb to work over the soft, puffy area on the inside edge of the foot. Then work along the ureter line up to the kidney. Always work on the inner side of the ligament line. Repeat on the left foot.

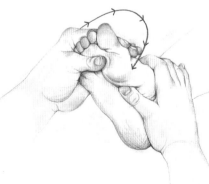

2 Work the kidneys

Support the right foot with the left hand. Use your left thumb to apply pressure to the kidney reflex and then rotate the foot around the thumb. (This way of working causes least discomfort in this very sensitive area.)

Treatments for enlarged prostate

Surrounding the neck of the bladder, the prostate gland is responsible for producing the fluid component of semen. When it becomes enlarged, as it often does in males over the age of 50 for reasons that are not clear, it impinges on the urethra, constricting and distorting it. Frequent urination, particularly at night when it disrupts sleep patterns, is common. Conventional treatment is either with long-term medication or surgery.

Reflexology treatment

So successful is reflexology in treating this condition that many patients who have received frequent treatments have ultimately found that surgery was not necessary.

Support Strategies

Kidney stones

Drink *at least 2 litres (3-4 pints) of plain bottled water a day.*

Diet *Eat a high-fibre diet low on animal proteins, both meat and dairy. Keep salt and alcohol intake down. Avoid sugars.*

Enlarged prostate

*A **natural progestogen** cream, or daily doses of zinc and marine fish/evening primrose oil, have had some success in causing this gland to shrink.*

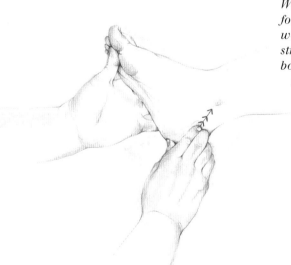

3 Work the prostate

With your left hand, support the right foot. Use your right index finger to work from the edge of the heel in a straight line up toward the ankle bone.

Repeat on the left foot.

Treating foot problems
Swollen feet/ankles, cold feet, chilblains

Restoring swollen/cold feet to normal

Sitting in one position for too long, as when travelling by air or on a long journey by road, may cause the circulation to become sluggish in the extremities. Immobility of this kind is one of the causes of swollen or cold feet. The problem is more likely to arise if you are pregnant, have varicose veins, or an old ankle injury.

High blood pressure, heart failure, or chronic kidney malfunction may also give rise to similar symptoms.

Reflexology treatment

As well as stimulating lymph drainage, reflexology treatment can help to relax the spine after hours of sitting.

Work first on the lung and heart areas to improve circulation. Both must be treated since their functions are so intimately connected. Then, since these organs are contained within the ribcage, work out the whole of the spine, concentrating particularly on the area of the thoracic spine, since nerves from this area send impulses to the heart and lungs.

If the feet are very swollen, treat the hands instead.

**Self-help:
working your own hands**

1 Work the heart *(see p. 37)*

2 Work the lungs *(see p. 32)*

3 Work the spine *(see p. 34)*

Memorize the above, then, if your feet are giving you problems on board an aircraft, you can get some relief by treating your hands.

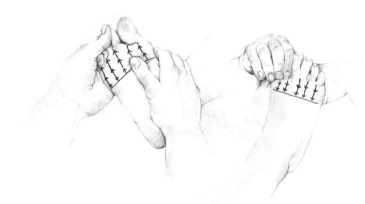

1 Work the lungs

First work the sole of the foot. Support the right foot with your left hand, and work up from the base of the diaphragm line to where the toes join the foot. Then work the top of the foot. First, make a fist with your left hand and press it into the sole to open the grooves on the top of the foot. Then use your right index finger to work down these grooves.

Repeat both procedures on the left foot.

Chilblains

Older people, in particular, are prone to chilblains, painful, itching, swollen areas of skin, usually on the feet, which are triggered by cold weather or a cold environment. Poor circulation, made worse in some cases by a poor diet, lack of exercise, and clothing that is not warm enough, leads the blood vessels just below the surface of the skin to constrict excessively in reaction to the cold.

Reflexology treatment

The aim of treatment is to improve circulation and it is the same as for swollen feet (left). If the chilblains are on the feet, treat the hands.

Support Strategies

Vitamin E supplements are beneficial for circulation.

Thick wool socks or stockings, as well as warm, lined shoes and slippers, help keep feet warm in winter. Avoid tight-fitting shoes that restrict circulation.

Lemon oil, applied locally, will give some relief from chilblains.

Avoid direct heat from open fires or hot water bottles if you have chilblains.

2 Work the heart

NB This reflex is found only on the left foot. Do not overwork it.

Support the top of the foot with your right hand. Use your left thumb to work the area in the direction shown. Do this for 2 or 3 times at the most.

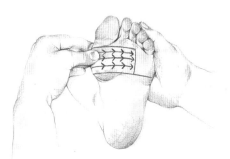

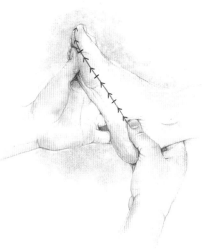

3 Work the spine

With your left hand, support the right foot. Use your right thumb to work the entire length of the spine reflex points, concentrating particularly on the thoracic spine area, midway along the foot.

Repeat on the left foot.

Allergic reactions

Common culprits: food sensitivities and stress

Almost any symptom that has failed to be identified as being caused by a specific disease can result from an allergy. This is an immediate or, more often, delayed physical reaction to one or more of a wide range of irritants or allergens. Physical reactions most commonly affect the skin and the respiratory and digestive systems. Irritants include certain foods, grasses, pollen, house-dust mites, animal fur, household sprays, and detergents – to name but a few.

Common symptoms of an allergic reaction, apart from the streaming eyes and nose usually associated with hay fever, are dark circles and puffiness under the eyes, chronic diarrhea, joint pains, headaches, and rashes, often with itching.

Food allergies

Sensitivity to food was first recorded by Hippocrates, who pointed out the link between milk and gastric upsets, and dairy products are now recognized as common allergens. Some physicians believe that sensitivity to food lies behind many undiagnosed aches, pains, and fevers. Allergic reactions to food are certainly implicated in a variety of common ailments, including asthma, rhinitis, runny nose, migraine, arthritis, depression, IBS, eczema, and psoriasis. You can identify culprit foods with an exclusion diet, and by keeping an allergy diary.

Heredity predisposes some people to allergies, though forms may vary. If there is a family history of allergy, mothers are advised to breast-feed babies for at least 6 months. Certain foods, including all dairy products, citrus fruits and other fruits with a lot of pips, and wheat products should not be offered until any baby at risk is a year old.

While attempting to identify the cause of a food allergy, it is important not to leave any foods out of the diet for very long (see the Allergy diary, right). It is certainly worth noting that many children who suffer from asthma have a less than average intake of

Allergy diary

To identify food triggers

Start by keeping a diary of your allergic reactions for a month, noting suspect triggers.

◆

For the next 3 weeks, stay 100 percent off the suspected culprit foods. Keep the diary throughout.

◆

Reintroduce foods one at a time, a week at a time. Take daily portions of the food for a week. If this does not trigger a reaction, keep it in the diet and try the next food. Keep on filling in the diary.

◆

When you have tested all foods, show your doctor your diary and ask for advice on future action.

Do not leave foods out of your diet on a long-term basis if their effects on your symptoms are not clear. Again, seek specialist advice.

vitamin C. It is important, then, to make sure that a young asthma sufferer has a healthy diet that includes a high proportion of fruit and vegetables, the latter preferably eaten raw.

The stress factor

Stress, which depletes the immune system, plays a major factor in triggering allergies. You may recall, for example, that at a particularly stressful period of your life you became allergic to the fur of your cat or dog, unusually sensitive to pollen, or whatever. At another period, the allergy seemed to disappear, or at least diminish. This was undoubtedly because the stress had also disappeared.

Reflexology treatment

Reflexology seeks to treat not the allergy itself but the reason why the body has developed the allergy. As well as encouraging deep relaxation, which helps dissipate stress, reflexology helps strengthen the digestive system. So, work the entire digestive system (see pp.100-101), concentrating on the liver, stomach, and intestinal areas. Work on the spleen to stimulate immunity (p. 31), and reduce stress levels with the relaxation treatments (pp. 24-25).

Suspect foods

Almost any food can cause an allergy. The list of prime suspects below may suggest a starting point in identifying culprits.

Wheat and wheat products

Yeast (in bread, cheese, alcohol)

Sugar

Milk and dairy products

Orange, red, and purple fruits

Food colourings and preservatives

Caffeine

Chocolate

Support Strategies

Cut out processed sugar. *The greater the build up of processed sugars in the body, the more an allergy thrives. Natural sugars, found in fruits, are not harmful in this respect, though some fruits provoke allergic reactions..*

Vitamin and mineral supplements *can be taken as long-term preventive measures Take 1g slow-release vitamin C daily. Take*

15mg zinc at night and a high-dose vitamin B complex (yeast free), once daily. Your urine will turn yellow if you are taking enough of the latter. If the allergy flares up, take 1g vitamin C up to 6 times a day.

Lower your risk *of developing a sensitivity by reducing to a minimum your consumption of refined and processed foods.*

Treating arthritis
Osteoarthritis, rheumatoid arthritis, gout

Pain, swelling, and stiffness in the joints result from the inflammation caused by one or other of the several forms of arthritis.

Osteoarthritis
In this, the commonest form of arthritis, the normally smooth cartilage in a healthy joint becomes rough and flaky. This means that the joint is less resilient and therefore more easily strained or damaged; the damage causes pain and stiffness. The problem, which affects the major weight-bearing joints, in the neck, lower back, knees, and hips, is exacerbated by wear and tear. Anyone over the age of 60 has probably got some degree of osteoarthritis, though it is not necessarily causing symptoms.

Sufferers who are overweight find that losing weight brings dramatic relief from symptoms.

Gout
This common joint disease is far more common in males than females, and can affect men at any time after puberty. Another form of arthritis, it is caused by excess uric acid in the blood stream, which leads to the formation of crystals of this acid in the joints. Unlike osteoarthritis, however, it tends only to affect one joint, usually the one at the base of the big toe. Affected joints become red, swollen, and so painful that the slightest pressue is unbearable.

Though some people suffer only one attack, most have had a second within 2 years. If you have had more than one attack, you are likely to continue to have them with some regularity. It is important to seek treatment after a second attack, since without it joints may become permanently affected.

Rheumatoid arthritis
One of the most severe of all joint diseases, this auto-immune disorder affects the lining of joints, which become inflamed and thickened, causing pain,

Treatment summary
including self help on the hands
1 The digestive system
(**F** pp. 100-101; **H** pp. 35-37)
2 The urinary system
the bladder (**F** p. 29; **H** p. 35)
the ureter (**F** p. 29; **H** p. 35)
the kidneys (**F** p. 30; **H** p. 36)
3 Work the appropriate reflexes for the affected areas
NB **F** = feet; **H** = hands

Keep the joints moving!
Hands: rotate the wrists slowly, first clockwise, then counterclockwise. Then wriggle the fingers.

Shoulders: rotate the shoulders in their sockets, first forward, then backward. Do this about 6 times both ways at intervals during the day.

Ankles: rotate the ankles clockwise, then counterclockwise, supporting the lower leg while you do so.

Support Strategies

Marine fish oils, or evening primrose oil, sources of esential fatty acids, help alleviate symptoms.

Cod liver oil is also helpful. Take 1 tablespoon mixed with 2 tablespoons of fresh milk,first thing every morning.

Cherries are said to prevent the crystallization of uric acid. Eat the fresh fruit, or drink the juice.

Cut out citrus fruits, meat, and eggs.

Start giving reflexology treatments – the exercise is good for stiff fingers and wrists.

Acupuncture has a considerable success rate in providing pain relief in arthritis.

stiffness, and swelling. It can affect any joint, but most commonly those of the spine, neck, shoulders, wrists, fingers, hips, and knees are involved. Ultimately, replacement hip or knee joints may be the only solution if damage is severe.

Reflexology treatment
The aim of treatment is to encourage the elimination of toxins, by working on all the organs of elimination in the digestive and urinary systems.

   In addition, work the part of the skeletal system that is affected – whether lumbar spine, shoulders, knees, hips or hands (see pp. 27-28 and pp. 33-35). Light massage of any painful part helps to improve circulation and the elimination of toxins, as well as to reduce swelling, giving more mobility and freedom in the joint.

Maureen, an elderly patient with arthritis

Since her late forties Maureen had suffered from arthritis, and over the years had resorted to anti-inflammatory and pain-killing drugs. But their prolonged use eventually led to a number of unpleasant side effects, including frequent digestive upsets.

When she first came to me, all the reflexes in her feet relating to the skeletal system were extremely sensitive, and I warned her that the treatment would probably produce a strong reaction. By the next day, she had developed a temperature, and ached in all her joints. A long-term sufferer from constipation, she also had attacks of diarrhea throughout the night. I welcomed these signs of a true healing crisis and was able to reassure both Maureen and her husband.

She went on to improve week by week and was eventually able to bend and pick something up from the floor – for the first time in years. The pain and stiffness in her hands reduced and she could move her neck from side to side. After 4 months she looked 10 years younger, her walking had improved amazingly, and she felt that she had been "reborn," thanks to reflexology. She continued with monthly maintenance treatments.

Chapter Five

Making Stress Manageable

Reflexology creates a sense of wellbeing, and this alone offers at least temporary respite from tension. Frequent treatments lead quickly to dramatic reductions in stress levels.

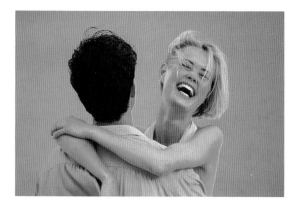

Taking time out *from the frantic pace of urban living, just to be yourself and recharge your batteries, is an essential part of keeping stress at a manageable level.*

Stress is unavoidable. You cannot escape it, though you may reduce its level by fleeing modern urban society and adjusting to the slower pace of rural living. Nonetheless you will inevitably have to face at some point certain life events, certain significant stages in your development as a human being that are recognized as being inherently stressful.

This chapter shows how you can use reflexology, in conjunction with other "support strategies," to make intrinsically stressful situations more manageable.

At the same time, reflexology can help reduce or dissipate the effects of long-term low-level stress. Start regular treatments at once if someone in your family is continually "stressed out." This kind of stress depletes the immune system, leading eventually to physical dis-ease – whether ulcers, colitis, or IBS – or depression and panic attacks.

The remarkably relaxing effect of reflexology enables people to begin to take charge of their worries, rather than being overwhelmed by them.

The abbreviations **F** (feet) and **H** (hands) are used throughout this chapter.

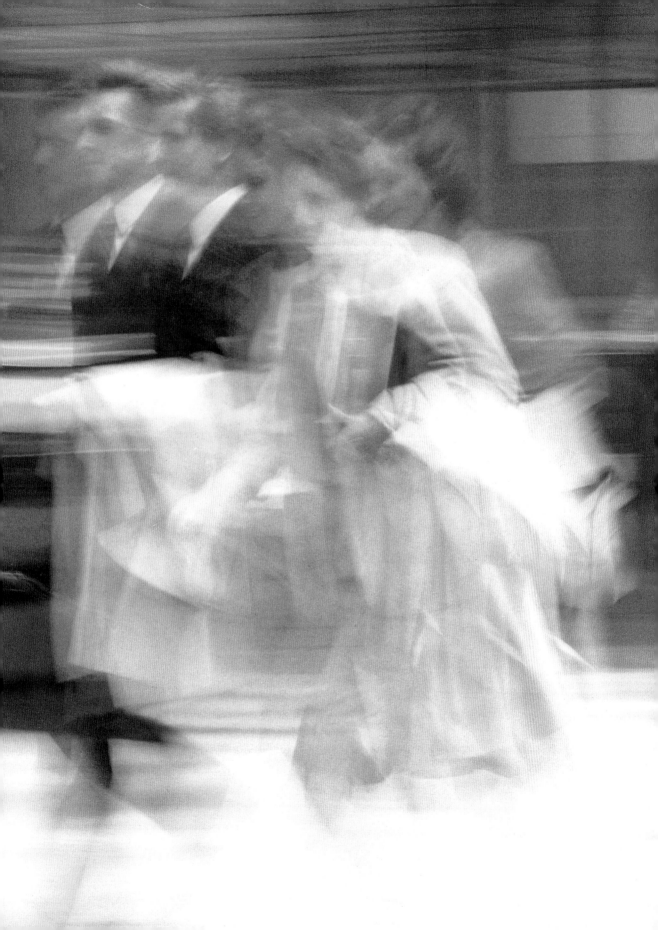

Restoring your inner balance

We are all human, and we all have our frailties. At one time we will be offering help, at another, receiving it. This section addresses the reader both as the giver and receiver of reflexology treatments.

Whether you work on your own hands or get a partner or relative to work on your feet, you are taking important steps to restore harmony and balance to your system.

Personal illness: a positive approach

Illness is physical or mental dis-ease. In order to remove this disease, holistic practitioners believe that it is essential to treat the whole person, that is, the mind and spirit as well as the body. Whether or not you subscribe to this belief, it is clearly sensible, if you are ill, to spend some time reviewing your physical and emotional life in order to establish whether there are steps you can take to ameliorate your situation in any way.

It is difficult for healing to take place if you harbour deep resentments about your illness. Trying to approach it in as positive a way as possible can have extraordinary results. Healers, for example, report on patients whose planned operations have not, finally, proved necessary: healing took place once the patient began to direct love rather than anger toward the problem area.

The role of reflexology
Consider your body as a sacred, living temple, to be respected and cared for. One way of caring for yourself is to work the hand reflexes related to your problem. This is an important self-help supplement to treatments on your feet and quickens your healing response. Consult pp. 32-37 for a complete hand workout that contacts all the same reflexes as in the feet.

Accidents as safety valves

Sometimes an accident or injury occurs when you have been overworking to an exaggerated degree. In such a situation, it may act as a safety valve.

It requires courage, but while you are "out of action" on one level, you can act very effectively on another. Decide to take responsibility for shaping your future the way you would like it to be, throwing out old, stultifying habits, resentments, and anger.

The role of reflexology
Accidents cause shock, and shock affects the immune system, so work the spleen reflexes, on the left foot or left hand, intensively (see pp. 31, 37). For breaks or injury to the hips, legs, or any part of the low pelvic area, work out the reflexes to the coccyx, hip, and lumbar spine every hour (see pp. 27, 33, and 34).

Support Strategies
Depression

Exercise! Regular exercise is an essential component of a happy as well as a healthy life. It raises the level of endorphins, natural "feel good" chemicals.

Eat a healthy balanced diet, low on fats.

St John's wort is a botanical medicine said to help depression. Take it as a tea or in tablet form.

Cut down/out nicotine, alcohol, so-called recreational drugs.

Cut out caffeine and chocolate.

Explore psychotherapy or counselling.

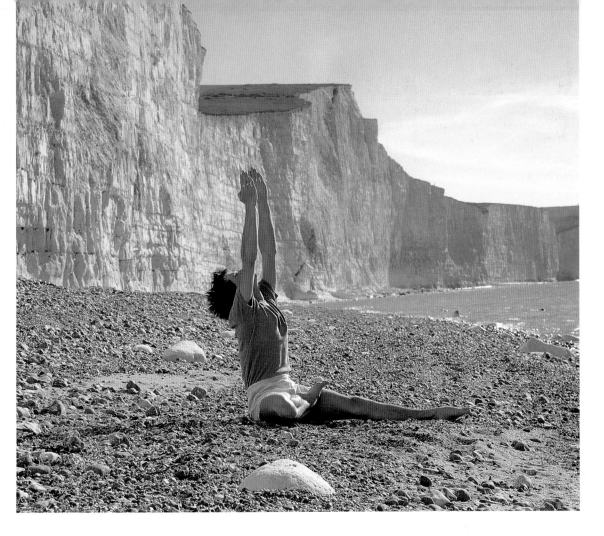

Depression

Every member of the family is bound at some time or other to suffer from depression – feelings of anxiety, sadness, and hopelessness. Such feelings may be a natural response to a particular event, but if the depression persists, or there is no obvious cause, it is more likely to be a depressive illness. Symptoms vary according to the severity of the illness.

Anxiety and mood swings are associated with mild depression; more severe depression leads to insomnia, tiredness, lack of interest in food or social activities, and loss of concentration.

Treatment varies: some people respond well to psychotherapy, others to anti-

"Opening up" postures in yoga, as well as the standing poses, are recommended for people feeling depressed. Strengthening and revitalizing, they discourage introspection.

depressants, yet others to a combination of the two.

The role of reflexology

Whether you are a teenager being buffeted by hormonal changes, a young mother suffering post-natal depression, an older man or woman going through a mid-life crisis, or are suffering from depression for no obvious reason, reflexology treatments can only improve your mood. As well as the healing power of relaxation, the treatment focuses on the endocrine system, since hormonal imbalances are frequently at the root of depression, and on the spine, to stimulate the central nervous system. Try to give treatments at least twice a week, in order to start giving relief as quickly as possible.

Treatment summary
1 Foot relaxation (see pp. 24-25)
2 Work the entire endocrine system (**F**: pp. 108-109; **H**: see pp. 108-109)
3 Work the spine (**F**: p. 27; **H**: p. 34)

Living through panic attacks
Overwhelming feelings of fear and anxiety, for no apparent reason, may strike someone out of the blue in a comfortable setting in which they feel perfectly at home. Panic attacks do not cause physical harm, and are rarely associated with serious illness, but they are deeply unpleasant and frightening.

Worries about breathing difficulty, sweating, trembling, palpitations, and a feeling of the "blood running cold" are typical symptoms. They are usually related to an anxiety disorder or a phobia.

Support Strategies
Panic attacks
Massage of the neck and shoulders with lavender oil may help reduce anxiety.

Regular vigorous exercise helps "burn up" the excesses of adrenaline that are released in panic attacks.

Meditation, practised regularly, eventually has a calming effect.

The role of reflexology
If you or one of your family suffer from panic attacks, try regular reflexology treatments to comfort them and induce a more relaxed attitude to life. In the midst of an attack, try to work on your own hands.

First, use all the relaxation exercises, then work the solar plexus and the entire spinal area to help the central nervous system.

Treatment summary
1 Foot relaxation (pp. 24-25)
2 Work the solar plexus (**F**: p. 93; **H**: p. 37)
3 Work the spine (**F**: p. 27; **H**: p. 34)

Getting a good night's sleep
Some people have difficulty going to sleep, others waken in the early hours and are unable to go back to sleep. Stimulants such as coffee, tea, or chocolate, undigested meals, and alcohol exacerbate the problem.

Family worries, about children and finances, about the state of health of aging parents, about your own or your partner's job security, all assume alarming proportions in the dead of night, making sleep impossible.But persistent insomnia is usually related to depression and anxiety.

The role of reflexology
The deep relaxation induced by reflexology should, if practised regularly, help break the pattern of sleeplessness. Use the foot relaxing routine (see pp. 24-25), repeating the diaphragm relaxing exercise 2 or 3 times, to induce sleepiness.

Disruptions to sleep patterns
The most common disruptions to sleep patterns are caused by jet lag and shift work. Long-haul eastward flights, that lengthen the traveller's day, tend to be worst for jet lag. Some people suffer from this so

severely that they make long air journeys only if essential.

People who do shift work and are constantly having to adjust to different sleeping and working hours suffer longer-term disturbances in the nervous system. Feelings of exhaustion, as well as, sometimes, nausea and insomnia are chronic features of their lives that inevitably eventually take their toll.

The role of reflexology
Reflexology can help regulate the body clock. The pineal gland at the base of the brain, often referred to as the "third eye," plays an important role in the adjustment of peoples' biorhythms. So, work the entire endocrine system (see pp. 108-109), concentrating particularly on the contact points to the pituitary and pineal gland, in the big toes. Balancing the brain area means that any overactivity is calmed down, and underactivity is stimulated.

A weekly treatment is recommended for people on shift work, in order to alleviate the stresses and strains of long-term disturbances to the nervous system.

Addiction 1: smoking

If cigarettes are the first thing you reach for in the morning and last thing at night, then you are addicted. As far as families are concerned, if one member is a smoker, the rest are too, passively – and the adverse effects of passive smoking are well documented. Subjecting your children to these risks is irresponsible.

Although the logic for giving up is overwhelming, you will only give up when you really want to – in your heart. You may arrive at this point overnight, apparently quite inexplicably. But your decision will probably be the culmination of long-term "interior" work, not even always on a conscious level. Once you have decided that you really do want to give up, reflexology can help by relaxing you.

Your self-image is more important than the one you project to other people. Learning to love and accept yourself are essential first steps if you are to stop destroying yourself. If your self-image is poor, seek professsional help in refocusing it.

The role of reflexology

The deeply relaxing effect of reflexology treatments should, over a period of time, reduce the number of occasions on which stress can provide an excuse to smoke a cigarette. All the family can participate in treating the smoker. Not only do they have a vested interest in living in a smoke-free zone, they can use the treatment times to express their loving concern for the smoker's health and wellbeing.

The aim of reflexology is not only to relax the patient, but to help repair the damage to those areas of the body most affected by smoking, that is, the lungs and heart.

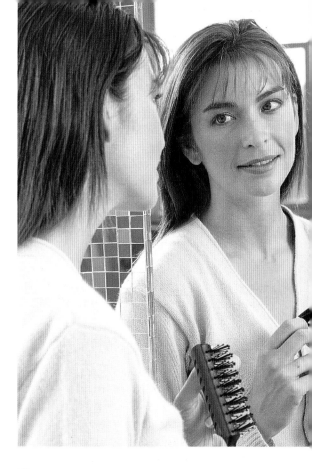

Treatment summary
1 Relax the diaphragm (**F**: p. 24)
2 Work the lungs (**F**: p. 26; **H**: p. 32)
3 Work the heart (**F**: p. 31; **H**: p. 37)

Support Strategies

Giving up alcohol

Accept help from your family, friends, or a counsellor. This is a first step on the way to learning to love, rather than destroy, yourself.

Join A.A. (Alcoholics Anonymous), who also run support groups for the families of alcoholics.

Acupuncture has a high success rate in dealing with alcohol addiction. Good results have been achieved through regular treatments over a 3-month period.

Addiction 2: alcohol

Persistent consumption of quantities of alcohol that exceed the recommended daily allowances is indicative of a dependence that needs to be recognized and dealt with.

The effects of alcoholism on the rest of the family, particularly if the drinker becomes abusive, violent, or incapable, can be devastating, and the help of an outside agency, such as Alcoholics Anonymous, is called for. However, as with any addiction, for such help to stand any chance of success, the addict first has to admit to having a problem and want, really want, to give up. Until he or she reaches that point, life for the family can be unmitigated misery.

The role of reflexology
As in the case of smoking, the reduction of stress is the primary function of reflexology. So use all the relaxation exercises. Then work the entire digestive system, concentrating particularly on the liver area. There is probably some degree of liver damage in any heavy drinker, and this will be evident in the sensitivity of the liver reflex.

Treatment summary
1 Foot relaxation (pp. 24-25)
2 Work the digestive system (**F**: pp. 100-101; **H**: pp. 35-37)

Eating disorders
Young people, girls and women in particular, conditioned by glossy magazines to equate female beauty and desirability with being thin, may become preoccupied with their figures, constantly dieting to lose weight. Some, for reasons that often are not altogether clear, are afflicted with an exaggerated and obsessive fear of getting fat: they then avoid food (anorexia nervosa) or indulge in binge eating followed by self-induced vomiting (bulimia). These potentially life-threatening conditions are deeply distressing, not least for parents, and must receive professional counselling and medical attention.

People who are grossly overweight because they eat compulsively also require professional help to identify the causes of their behaviour.

The role of reflexology
Reflexology can *only* be used as a back-up to professional treatment and counselling. The benefits of regular, healing, relaxing treatment will be appreciated not only by the patient but by the person offering it: parents, siblings, or partners often feel helpless when confronted by serious disorders in those nearest and dearest to them and are only too keen to do whatever they can to help.

Use all the relaxing exercises, then work the solar plexus and the entire digestive system. Work these areas regularly in an attempt to restore some balance. In addition, have recourse to one or other of the support strategies listed below.

Remember, however, that reflexology *cannot* take the place of essential professional medical help. Make sure the patient attends appointments.

Treatment summary
1 Foot relaxation (pp. 24-25)
2 Work the solar plexus (**F**: p. 93; **H**: p. 37)
3 Work the digestive system (**F**: pp. 100-101; **H**: pp. 35-37)

Support Strategies
Eating disorders
Daily exercise *(half an hour's brisk walking, for example) is good. Beware of compulsive exercising, which is often a symptom of anorexia.*

Eat regular meals*, sitting down.*

Don't go on fad diets! *All fad diets work and all fad diets fail, eventually.*

Feminist literature *may help some girls and women change their "mind set" in a positive way.*

Psychotherapy*, individual or group, may help get to the root of the problem.*

Yoga *tones muscles and increases body and self awareness, which may lead to increased willpower and the ability to resist the temptation to overeat.*

Babies and the blues

The decision to start a family is one of the most momentous a couple can make. As with any other of life's profound decisions, once made, it may bring its share of pain and disappointment as well as fulfilment.

Coping with postnatal depression

"Baby blues," usually starting a few days after the birth, affect two thirds of mothers, no matter how delighted and proud they are about the new arrival. Unpredictable tears, irritability, and depression are some of the symptoms, which usually pass within two or three days. These reactions, often unexpected, are primarily caused by sudden hormonal changes.

More severe postnatal depression affects some women, and may last for a period of several weeks or more, though it usually disappears of its own accord. The worst form of depression, which usually sets in about 2 or 3 weeks after the birth, is rare, affecting only one woman in a thousand. This is depressive psychosis and demands hospital treatment.

The role of reflexology
There are several levels on which the new mother can benefit from reflexology treatment. It can improve the functioning of the hormonal system, help alleviate discomfort in the vaginal and rectal areas, help relieve engorgement of the breasts (see also p. 91), and encourage a prolific milk supply.

Try to find an hour in the evening when the baby is settled and you – the parents – can have some time together alone. This is very important. Too often, fathers feel neglected by mothers who seem to have time only for the new baby.

Begin by giving the mother a complete relaxation treatment. Then work the endocrine (hormone-producing) system and the entire reproductive system. Working the latter stimulates nerve and blood supply to the vaginal area, which will improve muscle and ligament tone and assist the body in healing itself. Then work the area to the breast, found mainly on the top of the foot.

Treatment summary
1 Foot relaxation (pp. 24-25)
2 Work the endocrine system (**F**: pp. 108-109; **H**: see p. 108)
3 Work the reproductive organs (**F**: p. 30; **H**: pp. 36-37)
4 Work the breast **F**: p. 26; **H**: p. 32)

Boosting fertility and vitality

Many women feel that the ability to conceive and bear children is their birthright, and when conception does not to occur their

---

Support Strategies

To boost your fertility and vitality
Identify and take steps to reduce the impact of hazardous chemicals in food, water, home, and working environment

Learn to recognize, record, and interpret the natural signs of female fertility and time intercourse to maximize your chances of conception.

Cut out alcohol. Apart from anything else, it causes zince depletion which in men leads to reduced sperm count and reduced testosterone.

reaction is great frustration and sadness, perhaps turning to anger and even despair.

Medical tests are necessary to establish if there is any physical disorder preventing pregnancy and these are usually carried out if the woman has not become pregnant after a year of unprotected intercourse. If infertility is found in either partner, reflexology and other alternative therapies can be used to back up attempts at assisted pregnancy.

If no medical reason for not conceiving can be identified, there are numerous avenues to explore in order to maximize your chances of conceiving. Begin by eliminating possible dietary or environmental hazards that may be reducing your chances of conception. Research these yourselves or take professional advice.

Reflexology treatment
Start treatment at the same time as you embark on orthodox medical investigations.

While treatment cannot be proved to have contributed to conception, there have been many so-called "reflexology babies," conceived after 3 to 4 months of frequent treatment. Exchanging treatments between partners is recommended – each partner should receive treatment 2 or 3 times a week – but you also need to enlist the help of a professional reflexologist.

Treatment summary
1 Foot relaxation (pp. 24-25)
2 Work the hormonal system, particularly the pituitary and thyroid areas (**F**: pp. 108-109; **H**: see p. 108)
3 Work the ovaries/testes, prostate, and vas deferens (**F**: p. 30; **H**: pp. 36-37)

Laura and Simon: a fertility problem?

This couple had not married until their mid-thirties and were therefore disappointed when, after almost 5 years, a much longed for baby still had not appeared on the scene.

They both had all the usual tests, which revealed no abnormality. The only problem Laura had ever experienced was that her menstrual cycle had never been regular. Apart from that, her periods were pain free, and she enjoyed good health. Simon had never had any health problems. Keen to explore some form of complementary therapy, rather than resort to hormonal treatments that Laura was not happy about, they turned first to reflexology.

I decided to treat one partner one week, and the other the next, in an attempt to balance the weak link in the reproductive system which must have been there. The first sign of any change taking place was when Laura's monthly periods became regular, following a 28-day cycle, for the first time in her life.

I had warned the couple that any attempt at helping a fertility problem would mean several months of treatment. And I had advised them to abstain from alcohol and to take zinc supplements, as well as ginseng.

Only 4 months had passed when Laura telephoned excitedly to say she had missed her period. Two weeks later, tests confirmed that she was pregnant. Laura decided to continue with reflexology on a regular basis throughout her pregnancy, in order to keep her body in as healthy a condition as possible, and she came for fortnightly sessions.

She had a healthy pregnancy and an easy labour. Her new baby, Eleanor, was going to be introduced to reflexology at an early age.

Dynamic partnerships

Balancing the needs and energies of both partners is important if both are to derive equal satisfaction and pleasure from a relationship. This is not necessarily an easy task: it demands imagination, patience, understanding, and generosity of spirit.

Harmony in partnerships

Living intimately with another adult, sharing your space, time, and feelings with them on a day-to-day basis, usually means having to make adjustments and compromises that are not easy. Additional strains may be put upon a relationship by insecurity at work, often leading to overwork and fatigue, and worries about finance and the future. Such worries are common in the best regulated households and they ultimately create great stresses in a relationship. These may be expressed in angry reactions, or the anger may be supressed, leading eventually to depression and exhaustion.

The role of reflexology
Making a reflexology treatment once or twice a week part of your routine will boost both partners' capacity to put at least some problems in perspective. At the same time you both have a chance to relax and enjoy mutual caring, love, and esteem.

To create calm, use the diaphragm relaxation exercise. Work the solar plexus area to dissipate pent-up feelings. Then, since anger and emotional upheavals often lead to digestive upsets, work the entire digestive system. It is important that each partner gives and receives a treatment.

Treatment summary
1 Relax the diaphragm (**F**: p. 24)
2 Work the solar plexus (**F**: p. 93; **H**: p. 37)

3 Work the digestive system (**F**: pp. 100-101; **H**: pp. 35-37)

A healthy, happy sex life

People's sexual performance or desire may be adversely affected by a variety of problems. Most of these are partly or entirely psychological in origin, though some have a clear physiological basis. While the problem may be recognized by both partners, sometimes an individual harbours secret worries about their own, or their partner's, sexual response. It is important for both to recognize, discuss, and, if necessary, agree to seek professional help about such problems if they wish to resolve them.

The role of reflexology
Reflexology can make an important contribution in the case of the most commonly encountered difficulties: lack of

Support Strategies

Dance! *Many people find that dancing increases their sexuality and sensuality.*

Make a sensual sanctuary *of your bedroom, decorating and furnishing it in a way that makes it inviting.*

Seduce *your sensual selves in your private retreat, stimulating sight, sound, touch, taste, and smell, in ways you both enjoy.*

Make space *for sex or just for being alone for a weekend or even 24 hours.*

Mutual massage *with an aromatherapy oil can be relaxing or stimulating.*

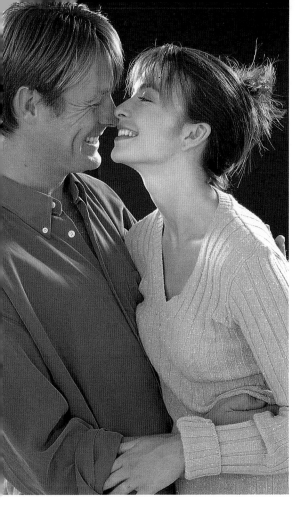

some of many possible contributory factors.

Never having been sexually comfortable, for psychological reasons, perhaps associated with a traumatic experience, is quite a different matter, which almost certainly calls for professional help.

The role of reflexology
The aim of treatment is to relax your partner and help dispel the anxieties which stifle sexual interest or lead to impotence. Work first on the solar plexus, the area that holds painful feelings: remember this may release powerful emotions. Then, to encourage total relaxation and lower the respiratory rate, use the general relaxation exercises. Finally, work on the genital areas.

Treatment summary
1 Work the solar plexus (**F**: p. 93; **H**: p. 37)
2 The foot relaxation exercises (pp. 24-25)
3 The genital areas (**F**: p. 30; **H**: pp. 36-37).

interest (which may affect both partners) and impotence in the man. While increasing both partners' sense of wellbeing, it allows them to share moments of quiet, tender relaxation in which they express mutual love and caring.

Touch, in this context, has more to do with sensuality than with the sexual expression of love. But it is every bit as precious and particularly important if it helps allay or remove fears and anxieties.

Reviving interest in sex
Temporary loss of sexual interest is likely to be associated with stress: young children, work, financial pressures, insecurity in the relationship, unresolved conflicts or resentments, illness, and depression are

Support Strategies
A loving approach to impotence
Explore other ways of enjoying sex. Penetration is only one way. Try touch, massage, mutual masturbation.

Talking openly about the problem, with your partner, counsellor, or friend, will help put it in perspective.

Certain drugs, including some used to lower blood pressure, cause impotency. Weight reduction has a good effect on blood pressure as well as on morale. If medication becomes a thing of the past, virility may return.

Accepting the end of an era

Change is inevitable, but it is not always easy to accept, particularly if it signals the end of an era. Be sensitive to the needs of people close to you when profound changes disrupt or threaten their familiar life pattern and they are thrown off balance.

Divorce and separation

This kind of loss may be almost as painful as bereavement, but rarely receives the same degree of sympathy or comfort. If children are involved, try to ensure that they do not assume any guilt or feeling of responsibilty for the break up of the relationship.

Reflexology treatment may be offered to children as well as adults and should follow that recommended for bereavement, p. 136.

Serious illness in the family

The onset of a serious illness or the result of a serious accident may change a normally healthy, active member of the family into one who needs constant care. If the illness imposes a significant change in lifestyle on all members of the family, it may mean that everyone has, to some extent, to adjust to the end of an era.

The more seriously affected patients are by their illness in terms of reliance on others for help with bathing, dressing, and so on, the more difficult it is for them to come to terms with their situation. This means that they require not only physical help but sensitive emotional support.

The frustrations of illness, leading to mood swings and irritability in the sufferer, often put enormous strains on the people who are caring for them. For this reason it is important to share the task of caring between all members of the family, allowing young and old to participate.

The role of reflexology

If the onset of an illness has created limited mobility, the patient may suffer from bowel problems (constipation) or even an infection of the urinary tract. Back pain and general stiffness result from lying or sitting for long periods. Reflexology can come to the rescue here, not only to improve bowel function, but to relieve stiffness, particularly in the lower back.

Take it in turns to give the patient daily treatments, until there is an improvement; then reduce the treatments to alternate days. Relief should be obvious in a short period of time.

Quite apart from the healing power of touch, the healing power of devotion will work positively for both receiver and giver. Children, particularly, are able to see that they have a contribution to make in a situation that otherwise might leave them feeling powerless and miserable.

Treatment summary

To improve bowel function:
1 Work the intestines (**F**: pp. 29, 31; **H**: p. 35)
2 Work the bladder (**F**: p. 29; **H**: p. 35)
3 Work the ureter (**F**: p. 29; **H**: p. 35)
4 Work the kidneys (**F**: p. 30; **H**: p. 36)
To relieve back stiffness:
Work the spine (**F**: p. 27; **H**: p. 34)

The menopause and beyond

When women move on past the cycle of egg production and uterus preparation, the resulting alteration in hormone levels in their blood is felt acutely by some. Hot flushes (flashes), memory loss, dry vagina, general aches and pains, and mood swings are experienced with varying degrees of severity.

Support Strategies

Sage, *in tea or tablet form, reduces hot flushes (flashes), as does bee pollen.*

Exercise *strengthens the bones and heart and promotes overall wellbeing.*

Cut out *smoking and cut down on drinking. You are at higher risk of osteoporosis if you smoke or drink more than 2 alcoholic drinks a day. And alcohol dilates the blood vessels, making flushes (flashes) worse.*

Vitamin C *is important for the maintenance of healthy bones. Take a 1g slow-release capsule a day. Eat fresh fruit.*

If stressed, take a high dose vitamin B complex, daily.

Eat *beans, pulses, and wholegrains, for protection against osteoporosis. Don't go overboard with dairy products for their calcium content, since your cholesterol level will go up. But don't use skimmed milk, as calcium absorption is poor – semi-skimmed is acceptable.*

In post-menopausal women generally, the loss in overall oestrogen and progesterone levels reduces protection from heart disease and can predispose some to serious thinning of the bones (osteoporosis).

Hormone replacement therapy (HRT) is helpful in reducing severe symptoms. It also offers increased protection against osteoporosis, and it *may* protect against heart attacks. It is not suitable for all women, however, and many prefer, anyway, to seek alternative natural methods of approaching menopausal problems.

Some of the strategies suggested for alleviating PMT (see p. 106) may equally usefully be employed to treat similar symptoms at the menopause.

The role of reflexology
The deeply relaxing effect of reflexology can be greatly beneficial in reducing feelings of stress and tension. In addition, working the endocrine (hormonal) system may help control hot flushes (flashes), which are caused by oestrogen surges. Some of the unpleasant symptoms of the menopause may be the result of chronic stress, leading to a serious depletion in the function of the adrenal glands (see below), so work on these is recommended. Complete the treatment by concentrating on the entire area of the spine, to stimulate the nerve and blood supply to the whole body.

Adrenal function
The stronger the woman's adrenal function, the easier will be the transition into the menopause.Excessive intakes of coffee and alcohol over a long period, chronic stress, and a poor diet all lead to adrenal exhaustion.If your adrenal reflex is very sensitive, you can be sure that your adrenal glands have been overworking for too long.

Treatment summary
1 Foot relaxation session (pp. 24-25)
2 Work the endocrine system (**F**: pp. 108-109; **H**: see p. 108)
3 Work the reproductive organs (**F**: p. 30; **H**: pp. 36-37)
4 Work the adrenal glands on top of the kidneys (**F**: p. 30; **H**: p. 36)
5 Work the spine (**F**: p. 27; **H**: p. 34)

Male mid-life crisis

Reduce your alcohol intake, if necessary. Excessive drinking adversely affects your performance on every level.

Diet A healthy diet (see p. 41) is a top priority for maintaining health and wellbeing.

Regular brisk exercise is essential for keeping muscles toned and weight down.

Handling the male mid-life crisis

It is now recognized that many men suffer from periods of severe depression starting in their mid to late forties. In extreme cases these may last for several years, and professional help, perhaps including a period of taking anti-depressant medication, is called for.

This is a period when some are subjected to extra pressures at work, since they are nearing the "top of the ladder," for others, it is a time for recognizing that certain ambitions will never be achieved. These stress factors, in tandem with questions about their virility, waning physical attractiveness, and the emergence of certain health problems, signal urgent action to avert an emotional crisis.

The role of reflexology
You cannot put the clock back, but there are a number of simple steps you can take to increase your virility, reduce your weight (if necessary), lower your blood pressure, and reduce your stress levels. A first practical step in this direction would be to get your partner to give you relaxing treatments, to

combat tension. Then work the spine, heart, and lungs to promote good circulation to all organs and functions of the body.

Treatment summary
1 Foot relaxation (pp. 24-25)
2 Work the spine (**F**: p. 27; **H**: p. 34)
3 Work the heart (**F**: p. 31; **H**: p. 37)
4 Work the lung (**F**: p. 26; **H**: p. 32)

"Empty nest syndrome"

This can affect both partners when the last child leaves home, to take up a job or go to university. Usually, however, it is the mother who suffers more: she may have devoted herself exclusively to bringing up the children, or combined the role of mother and wage-earner. She has probably been more intimately involved than the father, with feeding, nursing, nurturing, and counselling her offspring – and their departure leaves a big gap. The house seems empty and quiet. This, it seems, is the end of being needed.

If her partner is employed but she is not, the mother's feeling of loss may be acute, leading to deep depression.

The role of reflexology
Reflexology can be used in conjunction with a number of self-help measures that may enable parents suffering from "empty nest syndrome" to come to terms with their situation and exploit the freedom and opportunities it offers.

Exchanging reflexology treatments allows both partners the chance to receive and express affection, in a relaxed, gentle way. This can strengthen or revitalize a relationship that may have been neglected in recent years or overwhelmed by concerns about offspring.

If depression is a factor, consult p. 123 for

advice on specific reflexology treatments for this condition as well as on some helpful support strategies.

Allow yourself or selves to put your own needs first, perhaps for the first time in your life. It is very difficult to let children go, but try to trust them, and allow them to get on with their lives, while you get on with enjoying yours to the full.

Before you begin any relaxing work on the feet, give your partner a shoulder and neck massage, perhaps making it particularly special with your favourite aromatherapy oil (see p. 46) in order to help them to start unwinding. If there is time, give a full body massage.

Treatment summary
1 Shoulder and neck massage
2 Foot relaxation (pp. 24-25)

Cultivate your garden!

Do this figuratively as well as literally. Now you are both liberated from your immediate responsibilities to your children, you have the chance to devote time to yourselves.

Begin by paying extra attention to your diet and exercise – building toward a healthy old age. Then think about joining a society or club, studying for a degree, setting up a small business from home – whatever appeals to you – to fulfil your intellectual and social needs.

Don't limit yourself by "ageist" thinking, such as, "I'm too old to take up/do/go/start" whatever. It's your life, enjoy it!

Each generation, each individual brings a special contribution to the life of the family. Recognizing and prizing this leads to mutual esteem and dynamic, joyful interaction.

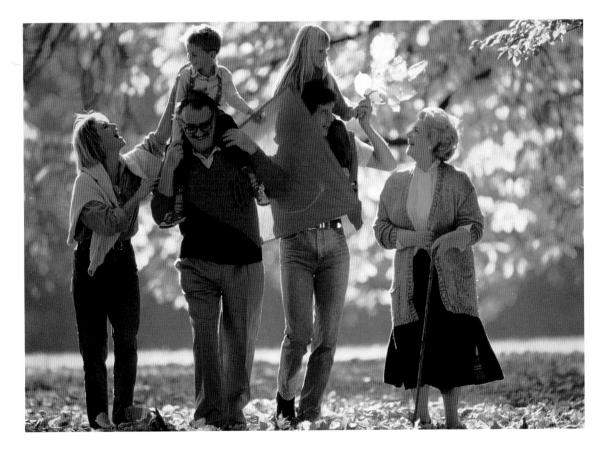

Terminal illness in the family

The awkwardness that many people feel in the presence of someone who is dying arises principally from the fact that for so long in the western world death has been a taboo subject. Now there are signs of change. People are beginning to reassess their approach both to their own death and to people who are dying. An important part of this is the recognition that if we deny death, we are unable to reach out to others, and they to us, at the very time when they need us most.

The role of reflexology
Reflexology is just one of several complementary therapies that families today can turn to for help in supporting a dying relative or friend as well as each other.

You may be at a loss for words – though it is important to let the dying person talk about their condition if they wish to – but you can say a lot, simply through holding someone. Physical contact is one of the most powerful forms of support you can give in the presence of pain and fear.

Use all the reflexology relaxing exercises on the feet (pp. 24-25). This will bring comfort and calm, perhaps inducing much-needed sleep. Let all members of the family offer this care.

Offer treatments only as long as the patient wants you to. And remember that someone who is very close to death probably wishes to be alone. Respect this wish. It is not a rejection of family and loved ones but a normal desire at this significant time of transition.

The death of a partner

When death is totally unexpected, shock makes it particularly difficult to accept. But even when it is expected, denial and hysteria are common reactions. There may be anger, too, directed at the doctor who was caring for your partner. Worse still, you may direct your rage at yourself for having, apparently, failed to do enough to help.

The real, deep sense of loss usually comes only after the funeral. The funeral arrangements, along with numerous other practical tasks, serve to some extent as diversions, certainly during the daytime. What is more, the bereaved person has been, up until that point, the centre of attention. Once the funeral is over, life for those less intimately connected with the family returns to normal. For the person who is left alone, the real pain is only just beginning.

The role of reflexology
People who have lost a partner need nurturing, and reflexology, offered when it

---

Support Strategies

Terminal illness

Pre-death grief unfolds in a similar way to bereavement, with denial, grief, anger, and resolution. Be aware of these states and respect them, in the patient and in yourself.

The holistic approach to caring for the dying may be one that you wish to explore – through books or appropriate organizations.

Be true to yourself at all times and sensitive to the real needs of the patient.

Support one another as carers. Make sure the principal carer in particular receives regular reflexology treatments.

seems appropriate at this difficult time, could be a very special gift. Enlist all members of the family in giving a treatment at least once a week, if wished.

Concentrate on the relaxation exercises, and spend some time working the spine reflexes on both feet. The latter will stimulate the nerve and blood supply to all organs of the body. End the treatment by massaging the soles, the sides of the feet, and the ankles with a soothing foot cream.

Treatment summary
1 Foot relaxation (pp. 24-25)
2 Work the spine (**F:** p. 27; **H:** p. 34)
3 Massage the feet with cream

Problems of advanced years

Not so very long ago, in the western world, if you reached the ripe old age of 70 you would be "doing well." Today, many people are living healthy lives way beyond that age. Keeping physically and mentally active, enjoying the company of friends and family, taking up the challenge of a new hobby or discipline – all are aspects of a positive, participatory attitude to life that can make your later years particularly fulfilling.

Nonetheless, most people are likely to suffer some physical discomforts as they age, particularly in joints that have been subjected to many years of wear and tear.

The role of reflexology
As well as helping to alleviate the discomfort of inflammatory or degenerative conditions of the joints (see p. 118), reflexology helps in pain relief through inducing a state of relaxation.

Treatment summary
1 Foot relaxation (pp. 24-25)
2 Work the spine (**F:** p. 27; **H:** p. 34)
3 Work the area affected by pain (see index)
4 Work the spleen, to boost the immune system (**F:** p. 31; **H:** p. 37)

Further Reading

Barlow, Wilfrid, *The Alexander Principle*, Victor Gollancz, London 1973

Ewards, Gill, *Living Magically*, Judy Piatkus, London 1997

Griggs, Barbara, *The Home Herbal*, Pan Books, London 1982

Holford, Patrick, *The Optimum Nutrition Bible*, Judy Piatkus, London 1997

Humphrey, Naomi, *Meditation: The Inner Way*, Aquarian, London 1987

Iyengar, B.K.S., *Light on Yoga*, Aquarian Press, Northampton 1997

Jackson, Richard, *Massage Therapy*, Thorsons, Northampton 1977

Jenson, Bernard & Bodeen, Donald, *Visions of Health*, Avery Publishing Group, Inc., New York 1983

Kabat-Zinn, Jon, *Mindfulness Meditation*, Judy Piatkus, London 1994

Kenton, Leslie, *Passage to Power: Natural Menopause Revolution*, Vermilion, London 1996

Lidell, Lucy, *Body Awareness: A guide to inner well-being*, Unwin Paperbacks, London 1987

Macrae, Janet, *Therapeutic Touch*, Penguin Books, London 1988

Maxwell-Hudson, Clare, *The Complete Book of Massage*, Dorling Kindersley, London 1988

Pearson, David, *The Natural House Book*, Conran Octopus, London 1989

Pitman, Vicki, *Herbal Medicine*, Element Books, Dorset 1994

Soo Chee, *The Taoist Art of Feng Shui*, Aquarian Press, Northampton 1983

Sivanda Yoga Centre, *The Book of Yoga*, Ebury Press, London 1983

Skynner, Robin and Cleese, John, *Families and How to Survive Them*, Vermilion, London 1997

Sutcliffe, Jenny, *Relaxation Techniques*, Headline Book Publishing, London 1993

Thomas, Sara, *Massage for Common Ailments*, Sidgwick & Jackson, London 1989

Tisserand, Robert, *The Art of Aromatherapy*, C.W.Daniel Co, Saffron Walden 1977

Walker, Peter, *The Book of Baby Massage*, Bloomsbury, London 1988

Worwood, Valerie Ann, *The Fragrant Mind*, Bantam Books, London 1997

Published by Gaia Books Ltd

Gillanders, Ann *Reflexology, A Step-by-Step Guide* 1995

Hayfield, Robin, *Homeopathy for Common Ailments*, 1993

Lavery, Sheila, *The Healing Power of Sleep*, 1997

McIntyre, Anne, *Folk Remedies for Common Ailments*, 1994

Mojay, Gabriel, *Aromatherapy for Healing the Spirit*, 1996

Stanway, Dr Penny, *Healing Foods for Common Ailments*, 1995

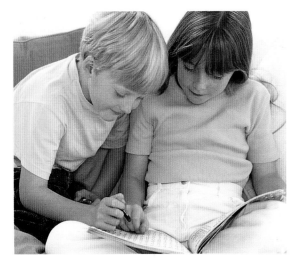

Index

Bold numerals refer to main text entries. Italic numerals refer to Support Strategies. **F** refers to foot; **H** refers to hand.

Acknowledgments

The author would like to
express her special thanks
to David King for all his
help, patience, and support
during the writing of this
book. Thanks, too, to Anne
Kilborn for her editorial
expertise, friendship, and
support, and to Phil Gamble,
for his sensitive, imaginative
design, and his unfailing,
good-humoured enthusiasm
throughout the project.

Gaia would like to thank the
following people for their
help in the preparation of
this book: Lynn Bresler (for
proofreading and indexing),
Jan Dunkley, Cristina Masip
and Michele Staffiero and
the photographic models:
Gemma Staffiero Masip,
April Bingham, Steve
Bullock, Suzi Perry, William
Flowers, and Steven Mills.

Photographic credits
Anne Kilborn p. 61
Telegraph Colour Library
pp. 38, 39, 44, 50, 51, 53, 65,
121, 120, 135
Special photography by
Annie Johnston pp. 2, 6, 7,
11, 21, 56, 72, 73, 126, 131
Iain Bagwell pp. 41, 47, 48
Andrew Rumball pp. 43, 123

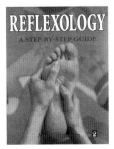

By the same author

REFLEXOLOGY:
A STEP-BY-STEP GUIDE
Ann Gillanders
ISBN 1 85675 081 7
£11.99

Reflexology: A step-by-step guide presents highly illustrated, step-by-step instruction in reflexology for selfcare and the care of a partner.

ALSO PUBLISHED BY GAIA BOOKS

TUI NA
Maria Mercati
ISBN 1 85675 038 8
£14.99 H/B

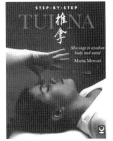

Step-by-Step Tui Na introduces the basic principles of this robust and vigorous massage which forms part of Traditional Chinese Medicine.

Now available with video -
ISBN 1 85675 069 8

Also available in paperback

NATURAL HOUSEKEEPING
Beverly Pagram
ISBN 1 85675 024 8
£14.99 H/B

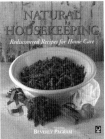

Natural Housekeeping rediscovers the recipes that kept households gleaming until chemicals invaded the home just a few decades ago.
Also available in paperback

NATURAL DOGS
Chris Madsen
ISBN 1 85675 048 5
£10.99

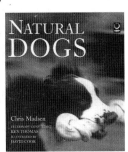

Natural Dogs provides clear guidance to understanding your dog and its basic needs for a health and happy life, with natural ways to treat ailments.

YOGA FOR STRESS RELIEF
Swami Shivapremananda
ISBN 1 85675 028 0
£11.99

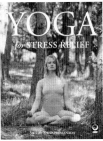

Yoga for Stress Relief offers a practical three-month stress management programme with step-by-step illustrated instructions and an explanation of the health benefits of yoga.

To request a full catalogue of titles published by Gaia Books please call 01453 752985, fax 01453 752987 or write to Gaia Books Ltd., 20 High Street, Stroud, Gloucestershire, GL5 1AS
e-mail address gaiabook@star.co.uk Internet address http://www.gaiabooks.co.uk